In a Moment's Notice

A Psychologist's Journey with Breast Cancer

Robin B. Dilley, PhD.

Publisher's Note:

This book is a psychologist's journey of awareness and healing that brings hope to those whose lives have been touched by a cancer diagnosis. It is intended to bring hope and inspiration for patients wrestling with life threatening illness and their families.

To engage the author to speak at your group or organization please contact her at drrobinbdilley@gmail.com or through her website at www.inamomentsnotice.com

Cover and Design by Roadrunner Printing, www.roadrunnerprinting.com

Photography by: RBJones photography, www.rbjonesphotography.com

ISBN: 978-1-456-31269-5

Library of Congress Control Number: 2011904549

Be patient toward all that is unsolved in your heart and try to love the questions, themselves.

Do not seek the answers which cannot be given you because you would not be able to live them.

And the point is to live everything.

Live with the questions now.

Perhaps you will gradually, without noticing it, live along some distant day into the answer.

(R. Rilke, 1934 <u>Letter to a Young Poet,</u> p.35)

Dedications

This book is prayerfully dedicated to

my loving life-partner,

Pam S. Smead,

for all of her support and love.

It is also dedicated to all of the strong women who have affected my
life and journey – especially my mother and Matt.

I also give thanks to my wonderful friends, colleagues, editors,
and supportive reviewers for their inspiration, encouragement and
insistence that I finish this book.

Foreword

Welcome to my journey with breast cancer.

In August of 1999, I was diagnosed with breast cancer. During that time, I kept a journal and copies of every medical record detailing the course of my treatment. In 2004 and 2005, I wrote about my journey, and then I put the manuscript in a box in my closet. The manuscript also lingered in multiple forms on various computers. In December 2008, I encountered another story when a mother of two adolescent boys died of stage four breast cancer. This death rattled me to my core. I knew deeply this woman's story, as well as many other stories of struggle, survival, and sometimes death. My manuscript began to haunt me from my closet. I dug it out of my closet and became friends with my story again. Today, I share my story with you.

It has been nearly eleven years since I was diagnosed and treated for breast cancer. Thus, in one sense, this foreword is a disclaimer. It is clearly a disclaimer about medical information. Breast cancer and its treatment have evolved over the past ten years in remarkable ways. The staging and pathology reports that I review now look very different to me from when I was dissecting and trying to understand my pathology report eleven years ago. The medical information in this book is only relevant to my story and my perception of my treatment for breast cancer over the last eleven years. This book is not intended to suggest any medical information for which you might make medical decisions. I hope what I have written will encourage you to ask questions, but please do not make your medical decisions based on anything I have written.

Throughout the book, I use real names of doctors and people most of the time. However, I have changed the names of some doctors and facilities. As you read the book, it will weave back and forth over the first five years during my treatment and then bring you up to date now eleven years later. I have attempted to make those chronological transitions easy for you to follow. I hope I have been successful.

My hope is that you will take away from this journey a well-told story that makes a difference to you in your daily life. If you or a person close to you is traveling this journey of breast cancer or any kind of cancer, my prayer is that my story will make a positive difference for you and bring a smile to your face while you grapple with your own journey.

Sincerely,

Robin B. Dilley, PhD.

How Dr. Dilley's experience can help you

When the cancer bombshell is dropped on a person, a number of things happen almost simultaneously. Each can affect the patient and those who are close to them.

One is the virtually inevitable sense of shock and the ensuing emotional roller coaster ride. Another is the delivery of a great deal of information by the doctor and being urged toward a course of action. Yet another is a flood of advice by well-meaning friends and family. Underneath it all is a pervasive sense of uncertainty.

Since nothing is really black and white and few guarantees are offered, there can be an incredible amount of stress for all involved. This underlying tension can persist throughout the treatment. Dr. Robin Dilley, in sharing her story, provides a refreshing sense of relief in a number of ways:

- She delivers hope. She is a cancer survivor and proves that cancer is not the death sentence it is often consciously or unconsciously perceived to be.
- She brings comfort. When you see her inner thoughts and feelings you know those you are experiencing are natural and okay.
- She avoids offering treatment advice; she simply relates how she arrived at the choices she made—which may assist you in making your own choices.
- She shares what she learned of her partner's experience as the one who went along for the ride but was not in the driver's seat.
- She gives solid, practical information on a number of unavoidable situations, like dealing with doctors, medical staff, and insurance companies.
- She details non-medical support resources she employed that can help you and your loved ones in working through your journey.

Perhaps the most important thing Dr. Dilley learned is that the patient is the only one in charge of their medical care. Knowing this along with the perspective Dr. Dilley provides can smooth the road for anyone dealing with a cancer diagnosis.

When Dr. Dilley received her diagnosis she desperately sought a book like this one to help her through. None existed then. One does now.

Table of Contents

CHAPTER 1

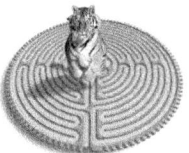

DISCOVERY

Silently gathering as social parasites attempting to take control of a perfectly healthy host, mutant cells slid into place, building a hard and ragged-edged dwelling on my right breast. Easily bored and thirsty for blood, they soon escaped their own space and dined their way into my lymphatic system, devouring healthy cells along the way. Now, drunk with their gluttony for power, they planned their next takeover. These mutant cells, not the smartest cells in my body, overlooked one small thing – *this* host notices changes in her body.

There it was pushing out of the skin on a hot summer day in July 1999, the weekend of July 16. I remember the weekend clearly because it was the weekend that the nation was captured by the minute-by-minute reporting of John F. Kennedy, Jr.'s plane crash into the dark, icy cold waters off Martha's Vineyard. I was lazing around, watching the story unfold, when my hand brushed across my breast, landing on a hard, zit-like bump. My internal sensors set off an alarm that produced a chill up and down my spine. I attempted desperately to shake this chilling fear and to lose myself in yet another Kennedy tragedy.

My attraction to the Kennedy family came from my mother, who idolized President Kennedy and wept tears of genuine pain after his assassination and during the public funeral. I knew if my mother were alive, she would be glued to the TV, just as Pam and I were on that hot July day. However, even the Kennedy tragedy could not shake the gnawing fear creeping up from my deepest place of knowing. I knew inexplicably that I, too, was being dumped into the abyss of a dark sea.

At first, I kept silent, returning in an obsessive way to touch and retouch that hard bump. Squeezing it, I soon discovered it was not a zit in birth. I was anxious, and the bump captured my concentration. Finally, my anxiety escaped. "Pam, do you feel anything here?"

She felt where my finger fit tightly over the bump, and said, "Yes, it's a small, hard knot."

Together, we monitored it while making inept attempts to encourage each other and drown ourselves in the CNN reports of the search for John F. Kennedy, Jr.

On Monday morning back at my psychotherapy practice, I called Ben Ora, a facility for mammography and ultrasound. I had chosen to have my mammograms at this facility because they used a special machine, lowering the amount of radiation my body received through the mammography. During that first mammogram there, Dr. Michelle West, a radiologist, pointed out that I had calcifications in each breast. "Lots of women have these. They are usually nothing to be concerned about, but we will keep an eye on them at your annual mammogram."

We had watched them for three years with no change. "I'd like to make an appointment for a mammogram with Dr. West," I told the woman scheduling.

"Do you have a prescription for a mammogram?"

"No, but I will get one as soon as I am scheduled."

"Was there any reason you need to see the doctor or is this just your routine mammogram?"

"Dr. West has been following my calcifications over the past few years, and I do have a small bump on my right breast," I said, as if it was nothing. "But it is time for my annual mammogram anyway."

"Dr. West's first available appointment is not until August 9, but Dr. Smith can see you next week."

"No, I don't want to see anyone else but Dr. West. I'll wait," I said.

I was comfortable with waiting. I knew I wanted to work with someone who I knew and trusted. Trust is the key for me. Receiving the diagnosis of breast cancer seemed like a very intimate thing, and I did not want just any stranger giving me the news. Besides, I was already busy: I had a trip to San Diego planned at the end of July, and was busily looking for and negotiating new office space. A month would give me time to monitor the bump to see if it had changed, even though I felt helpless to do anything constructive about it. Any information would be useful to the doctor and I knew one question would be, "Have you noticed any change since you discovered it?"

With the mammogram appointment made, I called Dr. Karla Birkholz, my primary care physician, to get the necessary prescription for the mammogram. Without a prescription, many insurance companies will not pay for a mammogram. I couldn't just walk in off the street and order my own mammogram in the same way I can't just walk into a laboratory and pay for my blood to be drawn. I needed a prescription or a written doctor's order to obtain my mammogram. Dr. Birkholz's office called me back to let me know they would mail it as I had requested. I recalled the scheduler saying, "Dr. Birkholz wants to know why you are waiting for a month?"

"It will be here before I realize it, and it is Dr. West's first available appointment," I said.

However, my nagging anxiety made me acutely aware that I was definitely waiting. But the mammogram appointment came soon enough.

CHAPTER 2

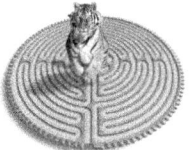

ENTERING THE SURREAL

I woke early on August 9, 1999 with a knot in my stomach. *Yep, this is it. It is cancer,* whispered the voice in my head, echoing through the depths of my belly.

The bump on my breast felt tiny compared to the desperation I felt. With unrewarded effort, I attempted to push it aside. "I don't have the facts yet," I told myself. "So just relax. There's nothing to be anxious about yet, except the squeeze of the mammogram."

Continuing my pretense that this day was just like any of the other 365 days in a year, I got up, dressed, went to work, and then went to my mammogram appointment just as if I was going to get my teeth cleaned. Just to throw in a little more normalcy, I also made an appointment with my attorney to sign the changes I had made in my will. I live in North Phoenix, and sometimes I treat going into downtown Phoenix as if it is miles away or a day trip. Thus, I had scheduled with Natalie, my attorney, on the same day as my mammogram appointment as a matter of convenience. Natalie's office was just around the corner from Dr. West's office. I reviewed my decision with a bit of amusement, though I'm sure I had not put together the idea that the process of updating my will might be necessary sooner than I had anticipated. Dying was not something that had entered my consciousness. How could one zit-sized bump on the outside of my right breast be lethal? That shows how little I knew about breast cancer at the time. On certain days, I yearn to return to that innocence.

In the waiting room, I distracted myself by thinking about the clients I would be seeing that day, mulling over their life scenarios and dramas. There are many advantages to being a psychotherapist; one of those advantages is dealing with other people's life dramas when I don't want to deal with my own. With just a tweak of the brain's focusing channel, I can leave my own story and enter another's. But the anxiety in the backdrop of my mind was overpowering and the refocus button just wouldn't work. The swirling in my stomach was like a dreaded roller coaster ride, an upside down nausea that knocked me off my feet as soon as I attempted to stand when the technician called my name.

Next, the tech asked, "Are you experiencing any changes in your breast?" That question interrupted my fog and I realized that I was in the mammogram lab with my top off. The morning and the drive to my appointment were lost somewhere outside of my awareness.

"Well it was time, I am due, but there is this bump that showed up in July," I said.

I showed her the bump and she positioned me to take several different breast images. With a quick exit and short return she came back and said, "Let me get just one more picture this way," as she pointed for me to step sideways. The large lump in my throat and the uncomfortable knot in my stomach competed for attention as I tried to focus and turned to my right. In her trained monotone she lied. "I'm just not sure how the last one turned out."

I have come to realize that technicians of mammograms, CT scans, and PET scans have a better ability to be stoic and expressionless at their jobs than I do at mine sometimes. She exited with her last picture and I re-robed and walked to the next waiting area. Soon Dr. West rounded the corner.

"How are you, Ms. Dilley? It's good to see you again." As I followed her back to her office, she began to tell me, "I've taken a look at your pictures. Let me show you what I am looking at and then we will do an ultrasound."

"Sure," I said nonchalantly despite my dry mouth and hard stomach.

We sat at her desk and looked at the images of my breasts on the special screen for viewing x-rays. She continued, "Here's your last mammogram. Here are your calcifications. Over here on this year's pictures, none of those calcifications have changed. However, right here –" she pointed with her pencil to the bump, "here is the problem. This looks very suspicious to me and I am eager to take a look at it on the ultrasound. How long has it been there?"

"Gee, Dr. West, it's as if it appeared overnight. I first noticed it on the weekend of July 16. It literally feels as if it just appeared out of nowhere on that day. But there has been no change in it over the month." I said that last sentence, offering my best words of self-encouragement.

"Well, let's take a closer look."

We moved to the ultrasound room. I lay back and put my hands behind my head. She examined both breasts and spent some time walking her fingers around the bump. She opened the container of cold gooey gel and placed it on my breast. This cold goo helps the ultrasound device smoothly explore the breast area.

The best thing about the ultrasound was that I could watch the screen as she explored my breast with a device that looked like an adjustable showerhead. My breast tissue appeared to be very much like the landscape of the moon – dark, and full of crevices. I amused myself by imagining that I was moonwalking on them. However, the truth is that I wasn't watching the ultrasound as much as I was reading Dr. West's face, serious and intense as she explored the images on the screen. She went over and over the bump as if she was trying to erase it, like the motion of cleaning off a blackboard. Finally she said, "It's this area right here. All of this area is smooth and here we can see the intrusion into the layers of the breast."

"Yeah, I can see it there," I said in a monotone.

I was entering that deep space inside of myself where I hide when the lights are going out in my world. When I'm in this space, I am calm on the outside, in control, undaunted, poised, and give no indication to anyone how I am reacting to the information I am being given. Her voice reminded me of a weather warning: "A storm front is moving in. Winds will be gusting to fifty miles per hour and a severe thunderstorm advisory has been issued."

I like having this interior space. It helps me feel safe. I cry over stupid things, like the singing of the National Anthem, sports wins and losses, a commercial featuring a parent and a child, or that damn Boston terrier commercial. I am always amazed at the silly things that bring tears to my eyes. But when the chips are down and the next poker move is mine, no one can read me. That's the way I want it. Dr. West finished the ultrasound and I sat up.

"Ms. Dilley, this does not look good. I don't know if it is cancerous or not but I want it out immediately. It certainly has suspicious characteristics. Who's your doctor?"

"Dr. Birkholz is my primary care physician."

Dr. West continued to stress how quickly she wanted this growth out of my body. Dr. West said, "I want this out of your body immediately! This growth is not something I want to just follow and see if it changes." In the next breath, she attempted to reassure me as well, saying, "Even if it is cancerous, it's so small that you'll be fine. You found it very early and due to its size it is very unlikely to have traveled anywhere else in your body."

There was something convincing in her voice. I am going to be fine. This really is no big deal. It will be no worse than having a root canal, my mind babbled.

It was not only Dr. West who said, "It's so small, you'll be fine." Later my surgeon would echo those same words. Even during my first oncology visit, my oncologist seemed riveted by the smallness of the lump as he read the pathology report. That was until he got to the bottom page of the pathology report. Everyone hoped and believed that because the bump was so tiny there was almost no way cancer could have traveled to my lymph nodes.

I finished with Dr. West, and paid my $25 co-pay as if everything was business as usual. I got in my red Jeep Cherokee and pointed it in the direction of Scottsdale Fashion Center. Pam's birthday was only ten days away and I still had shopping to do. Just for a moment the thought crossed my mind, *I wonder if I will be celebrating her birthday next year.*

I dismissed it, banning it from my consciousness, and called Pam on my cell phone. Using my cell phone while driving is a bad habit that I no longer practice, but the technology was so new back then that the convenience of having immediate access obstructed my common sense. "Honey, Dr. West does not like the way it looks. It is hard and has an odd shape. Dr. West is going to call Dr. Birkholz and I will have to make an appointment with a surgeon. She thinks it needs to come out right away but that there is not much to worry about because it is so small."

I pretended not to be scared since it was "so small." Pam followed my lead and also pretended not to be afraid. By the time we were finished talking, I was at Scottsdale Fashion Square Center.

"Got to go," I told her. "Call you when I get back in the car. I'm doing a little shopping for your birthday. I love you."

"I love you, too. You will be okay. Don't worry, honey."

I took an extra twenty minutes while Dillard's wrapped the presents to sneak into a bookstore. I headed to the health section and found a few books on women and breast cancer. I saw a big fat pink and white book by a Dr. Susan Love on breast cancer. I picked it up and scanned its pages full of information on types and stages of breast cancer. Then I put it back on the shelf. "I don't need this yet," I told myself.

Then I picked it up again, stared at it and put it down again. Again, I affirmed to myself, "I don't even know yet if I have breast cancer, so don't go borrowing trouble."

But in that small dark space inside of me a scream echoed from hidden chambers: *You know what you know, and this is not good.*

I left the bookstore in a panic and went back to pick up the beautifully wrapped packages.

Traveling back to my office with presents in tow, I tuned in to National Public Radio, because there I could lose myself in some world trauma. Checking my messages back at my office, only three hours after leaving Dr. West's office, I played back a message. "Robin, this is Karla Birkholz. Please call me and have me interrupted as soon as you get this message."

Even though my next counseling appointment was sitting in the reception room, I still had ten minutes before I needed to open the door and start the session. Picking up the receiver, I nervously dialed Dr. Birkholz's number and interrupted her patient care as she had requested.

"Hey, Karla, this is Robin," I said in my best chipper voice. She didn't even acknowledge that I spoke.

"I received a very distressing call from Dr. West."

Who was distressed, I wondered, *Karla or Dr. West?* After all, I was not. I had been shopping and finished all of the final details for Pam's birthday.

"Dr. West tells me this tumor is probably malignant based on its shape and she wants it out right now."

What I wanted to say was, "Sure, I've got this X-acto knife in my desk drawer. I'll just cut it out right now. It's so small; I can put a Band-aid on it."

But I said nothing and listened, though the next question seemed just as silly. "Do you have a surgeon?"

Sure, I have one in my back pocket, I thought. "No, I haven't had any surgery since I've lived in the Valley."

"Well, if it's okay with you, I will have my scheduler call Dr. BW. I've known him for a long time and I think he will be a good choice. I'll have them make the first available appointment for you."

Man what a bother, I thought. *My schedule is going to be interrupted with all of this.* "Okay, make the appointment, let me know as soon as it's made so I can move my schedule around," I said.

Within just three short hours my bump lost its status as a bump and was now being renamed a tumor. I wondered, *Don't bumps need to be larger to be called a tumor?* I quickly dismissed the word as medical jargon. Dr. West had only referred to it as "it."

I looked at my watch. It was 3:00 p.m. straight up. I opened my office door to my next client. "Hi, are you ready?"

I was surprised that I was able to concentrate on a word coming out of my client's mouth, but I was thankful to hide in someone else's misery.

My tumor would still be there when I finished the session.   Until this big crisis, I had never really realized what an escape my job was from my own life.

By the time I checked voice mail again, I was scheduled to see Dr. BW on Wednesday, August 11, 1999. The information and urgency of the newly-developing medical crisis were quickly sinking into my consciousness. The blur of the book with the pink and white text fought for my attention. I could see it swirling around in my mind's eye. I called Pam on the way home and said, "I'm going to swing by Borders and pick up a book I saw earlier today."

"Which book was that?"

"I can't remember its name or author, but some huge book on breast cancer. It was pink and white.   I imagine it has a lot of useful information in it for us."

"Okay, honey, but be home soon." I detected the worry in her voice. We both were buckling up for a ride that neither of us had chosen.

That evening we talked and read many, many pages of **_Dr. Susan Love's Breast Health Book_**. Pam and I found our way over to Chapter 19, "Understanding Breast Cancer."   We read with hope on page 269, "Most people believe that the size of the tumor alone determines its severity. Generally speaking they are right."

However, Pam and I missed the first sentence of that paragraph: "… at this point we come up against another misconception."

We read about the types of breast cancer, such as infiltrating ductal, invasive lobular, and inflammatory, noting many other types. We began to formulate some questions: How will we know exactly what type of breast cancer it is? How will we know if it has spread to other parts of my body? What will be the best route of treatment? What is the most aggressive treatment?

These questions sounded simple to us in our current state of naiveté.

CHAPTER 3

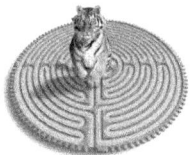

THE MUMBO-JUMBO OF THE NEXT WEEK

Tuesday passed like any other day, and on Wednesday, Pam and I took our first trip to the surgeon. The only surgery that I had ever had was arthroscopic knee surgery in 1987. Compared to cancer, knee surgery just doesn't feel like it counts.

Pam and I had discussed how we wanted to address our same sex relationship prior to the visit. We discussed in detail the biases and prejudices surrounding gay and lesbian people. She offered me the option of introducing her as my friend. I would hear nothing of the sort. I am who I am, and I was not going to start an arduous medical journey by making any attempt to keep a secret. I was accustomed over the years that we have been together of placing her as my person of contact in the medical informational sheet. In the space that follows "Relationship?" I always put the words "domestic partner."

When Dr. BW entered the room, he introduced himself and shook hands with each of us; I introduced Pam saying, "This is my partner, Pam." He showed no sign of discomfort and shook Pam's hand. He then pulled up a doctor's stool and began to ask some questions of both of us, including Pam in our discussion.

After looking at the film from the mammogram, he examined my breast. Then he drew us some pictures to explain the tumor. "Here in this left corner is the tumor location. It is tiny for a tumor. In all likelihood it has not traveled over here to your lymph nodes."

He said this while demonstrating with his pen. Two days into this, I knew hardly anything about breast cancer, but I knew enough about my body to understand that the lymph nodes are the gateway to and from the immune system.

"We want to remove it immediately, and see what the biopsy tells us. When we get those results we can talk about your options," he said. We concluded the appointment and followed him down the corridor to the scheduling desk.

He told the scheduler, Heather, to schedule me for the first available surgery slot. The first available time was the following Monday, August 16. Heather went over my instructions for pre-operative preparation: nothing to eat or drink after midnight, be at the hospital two hours early, and bring my insurance card with me.

The weekend arrived and Pam and I searched the web for information on breast cancer. We typed "breast cancer" and pushed the search button. We found 1,978,000 sites. That was in 1999. In January 2010, I entered the same two words and 38,500,000 hits appeared.

"Well, we can make a lifetime of research out of this. Where do we start?" I asked Pam.

We decided that the logical places to start were the American Cancer Society, The National Cancer Institute, and the Susan G. Komen sites. Susan G. Komen has become a household name for breast cancer research. It is the largest and most visible organization providing hundreds of millions of dollars to breast cancer research and prevention programs. The Susan G. Komen foundation began as a promise between two sisters, Susan Goodman Komen, and her sister, Nancy Goodman Brinker. Susan was diagnosed with breast cancer in 1978 at the young age of thirty-three. She died three years later at the age of thirty-six, after fighting a courageous battle against the disease that assaulted her body.

Before Susan's death she asked her sister, Nancy, to do everything she possibly could to find a cure for breast cancer. Nancy kept her promise and today the Susan G. Komen foundation has more than 100,000 volunteers and the largest series of 5K runs that generate millions of dollars of revenue. These dollars provide innovative research and community-based outreach programs, fund research grants, and support education, screening and treatment projects within communities. Pam and I felt comfortable researching the Susan G. Komen site because we believed it would be politically unbiased and it was really the only name we knew in relationship to breast cancer.

The first rule in research is to go to what you know before you branch out into unknown territory. We still didn't have enough information to do an in-depth search, not knowing what type or what stage of breast cancer I had. In that dark space that I keep referring to, I secretly nursed a bit of hope that this tumor was not malignant at all. I knew I was not being realistic. But, despite my internal awareness, I reminded myself, "They don't know yet, really. There is no pathology report."

Even without the specifics about the nature of my tumor, Pam and I managed to spend all day Saturday and Sunday on the World Wide Web trying to grasp some sense of personal control, to gain a helpful arsenal for our questions, and to distract ourselves from that eerie, creepy, angst that was settling into our daily awareness. The words "breast cancer" were not supposed to be rolling off of my tongue about me. This was something that happened to other people. The research gave us something to do while we each worried in our own way.

Our anxiety took over sufficiently, so we could no longer drown ourselves in TV or movies. The John F. Kennedy, Jr. story was over. There was no current national tragedy, no exciting sports, or anything to help distract me. I discovered that when I sat in front of the TV to watch CNN, I could not recount one single story or headline fifteen minutes later.

Pam and I topped off our weekend by going out for Mexican food and drinking margaritas. The margaritas took the edge off and pushed the anxiety back to a manageable space. What was going to happen? Was I going to have to have chemotherapy? Would I throw up? Would it hurt? Would I lose my hair? Would I live?

CHAPTER 4

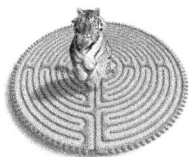

THE BIOPSY AND A LOOK AT RECONSTRUCTION

Monday, August 16, just seven days after the bump had been declared to be a "tumor," I arrived at the hospital unfed and ready for my biopsy.

The first part of my biopsy was of the calcification. According to Dr. Love's book, this was called a *core biopsy*. I was fully awake for this and I firmly believe the medical profession seriously needs to consider another perhaps more sophisticated way of going after this calcification. I saw pictures of this procedure in Dr. Love's book. I knew I would lie face down on a cold table and my breast would hang out a hole. I found myself wondering if my breast was really big enough to hang down through that hole, or hang anywhere for that matter. I am small-breasted.

Dr. BW climbed under the table and squared off my hanging breast. In my sick sort of humorous way, I envisioned a car mechanic, "Yep, I am under here, trying to figure out what the problem is. Is it the alternator? The heat pump? What's the problem?"

My fantasy of the car mechanic dimmed as the large needle was inserted into the circled calcification marker. "Ouch!"

I held my breath for what seemed like hours, but in reality was only seconds, as the needle left its sting and extracted breast cells for the pathologist. A local anesthetic helped to numb the skin where the needle went in. Once in the breast, it was a different matter. Obtaining a sample of these cells was crucial to the pathologist. The calcifications seemed to be the most suspicious culprit, feeding the teeny tiny tumor.

I shuffled down from the cold steel table and climbed onto another gurney to be wheeled into an operating room. They removed the lump without any help from me and sent it off to pathology.

On Wednesday, August 18, I went to Dr. BW's office for the results. No one gives results over the phone, which has its upside and downside. The upside is that you have your doctor's undivided attention to ask as many technical questions as you would like. The downside is the waiting. The waiting game throughout these past years has been the hardest for me.

Dr. BW entered, and after going through the polite hellos, said, "The tumor is diagnosed as a ductal carcinoma. It is less than one centimeter in size. It is estrogen positive."

"What's estrogen positive?"

"It means the tumor was fed and kept alive by your estrogen. That's not particularly a bad thing. We have a drug called Tamoxifen to treat that. Let's take a look at your options."

He pulled out more paper and drew more pictures. He was not particularly artistic, but good enough for me to get the picture. "You can have a lumpectomy, which in this case would be going back to get any margins left behind in the biopsy. However, the statistics on lumpectomies show a higher recurrence rate than a mastectomy. Either way, I will need to take some lymph nodes."

Today the medical profession has a better way of taking lymph nodes, a procedure called a sentinel node biopsy.

"The biopsy of the lymph nodes will let us know if the cancer has spread to other parts of your body. Once again, I seriously doubt it, due to the fact that it is less than a centimeter. That size makes it highly unlikely that it has escaped its site."

Dr. BW continued, "If you choose to have a mastectomy instead of a lumpectomy, you will reduce your chances of recurrence. Regardless, you are premenopausal and you will need to have at least four rounds of chemotherapy. That is the standard of care for premenopausal women."

Pam and I had already discussed my options and agreed that I wanted to take no chances and be as aggressive as possible. A mastectomy is a hard decision for many women to make. However, the decision between playing around with odds that statistically showed recurrence versus having a mastectomy seemed quite easy. It was not a flippant decision —"Cut it off because I don't need it anyway"— but a somber and sacred one that would help save my life.

I said, "Dr. BW, Pam and I have already discussed this. I decided before I came to your office today that if this tumor was malignant then I want a mastectomy."

"I think that is a very wise decision, Robin. Do you have any interest in reconstruction? If you do, I'd like to have the plastic surgeon do the reconstruction at the same time as the mastectomy. I want to schedule the mastectomy right away."

"I doubt it, but how would I proceed if I want to check out that option?"

Pam and I had also read quite a bit between doctor appointments about the reconstruction options. In 1999 my reconstruction options were either a saline implant or a TRAM (transverse rectus abdominous muscle) flap. The TRAM surgery concerned me because of the amount of surgery required to cut stomach muscle, veins and blood vessels and push them up to my chest to make a breast. Strange and sometimes humorous things bother us at the weirdest times. For instance, even though I am not very athletic, I like to pretend I am and my understanding of the TRAM flap was that my stomach muscle would be compromised for the rest of my life. I was already giving up my breast. Did I also have to choose never to do another sit-up at this time? Of course, I can probably count on my left hand how many sit-ups I have done since August of 1999, but some things seem important at the time and later a different sort of perspective takes shape. Jacquelyn Kennedy Onassis said something along the lines of, "If I had known it was going to end up like this, I would not have done so many damn sit-ups."

Thus, the saline implant really was my only consideration at the time.

"Heather can set you up an appointment with a plastic surgeon. We use Dr. Smith. He's here in this building and does a nice job. Heather can see if he's on your insurance plan and set up an appointment if you would like."

Pam and I looked at each other. "Sure, that will be fine."

I was quickly scheduled to see Dr. Smith that afternoon. Heather also scheduled the mastectomy for Monday, August 24.

Pam and I had a rather quiet and somber lunch and returned to Dr. Smith's office. We were greeted by his petite slender office assistant and escorted to a private room where we were given a portfolio of information about reconstructive breast surgeries. "Here, take a look at these and Dr. Smith will be in shortly," she said.

Pam and I began to flip through the book. I quickly noticed that I could still see a residual scar in the photos. I had already tapped into significant emotional material about the scar that would be left behind. Losing a breast was one thing, but the thought of looking in the mirror and seeing a reminder scar was difficult to assimilate. I understood that

I would have a scar from under my armpit all the way across my right chest wall. Looking at these pictures did not take that fear away.

Dr. Smith entered and introduced himself. "These look very nice; however I can still see the scar," I said.

"That fades with time."

"Does it ever go completely away?"

"No. I want to be candid with you. Our practice of medicine is in many ways still very archaic. The scar will never go completely away. What I do is insert an inflatable breast shape into your breast area at the time of your mastectomy. After you begin to heal from the mastectomy, you will come to my office weekly and I will expand the breast slightly each week with saline solution. When we have it the matching size of your other breast, we tattoo on a nipple."

"I want some time to think about this and talk it over. If I choose to have the reconstruction, are you flexible enough to do it next Monday the 24th? Dr. BW's office is scheduled for that date."

"You make a final decision and Dr. BW and I can work out our schedules," he said.

By this time, I was so emotionally exhausted with all of the research, options and information coming at me I had very little politeness left. I was beginning to show wear and tear from trying to process so much information. I was aware that my current medical team seemed to be moving at a rapid speed – a speed that I didn't think was possible within the medical field.

Today, I hear horror stories of women waiting weeks to obtain a mammogram and weeks to receive their results. When something is wrong, it's often a very long process to reach a diagnosis. However, the express speed of my own diagnosis left me little time to absorb all the information and I was feeling confused.

 I knew I needed to gather more information. I did not want to make a major decision for reconstruction in just a few hours. That evening I called a woman from Bosom Buddies to discuss my options. I had never met this woman, but an amazing thing happens when you are diagnosed with cancer. A network of people – angels, really – appears out of nowhere to come along beside you to help you with questions and concerns. After I hung up the phone, I decided to give my body all of its resources to fight the cancer. I did not want it to have to fight off the foreign object in my body called a saline implant. Consequently, I chose not to pursue reconstruction. Now on the days that I need to wear a bra, I wear a prosthesis. However, I find the word prosthesis to be much too sterile to describe what I affectionately call my *mail-order tit*.

CHAPTER 5

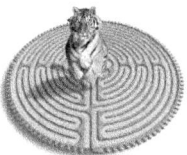

INFORMING MY CLIENTS

For about nine days I functioned at my office as if everything was normal. However, after the biopsy confirmed that yes indeed I had cancer; I knew it was time to start informing my clients.

I looked in my appointment book and allowed the face of each client to enter my consciousness. Each one trusted me with the most intimate details of their lives. Telling them was going to be tough, but only fair to them.

It has been proven that the relationship between the therapist and the client is the most important ingredient in good psychotherapy. Most clients come to therapy with some sort of attachment disorder covered over with layers of shame. According to master therapists like Carl Whitaker, Murray Bowen, and Virginia Satir, there is no such thing as a family secret. I teach students what I believe to be true from those master teachers: at some level within every family member there resides a seed of truth. Young children may not be able to articulate it, adolescents may act it out, or parents may fall into the same patterns of denial as their parents did, but at some level everyone knows "something is amiss."

I knew my clients would be able to tell, if they had not already picked up on it, that the atmosphere in the office had made a subtle shift and they would soon discern that "something was amiss."

Developing an attachment with one's caregiver is a key developmental task that can have several implications throughout life. Inadequate maternal care during early childhood can have adverse influences on personality development. Attachment itself is a reciprocal, enduring emotional tie between an infant and a caregiver, each of whom contributes to the quality of the relationship. Attachments have adaptive value for babies, ensuring that their psycho-social as well as their physical needs will be met. According to ethological theory, infants and parents are biologically predisposed to becoming attached to each other, and attachment promotes a baby's survival. No other variables, it is held, have more far-reaching effects on personality development than do a child's experiences within his/her family. When a client enters psychotherapy, the client must develop positive attachment to the therapist in order for the client to heal old wounds, especially attachment wounds.

My developing a life-threatening disease would have an emotional impact on my clients, an impact for which they had not signed up. There are no hard and fast guidelines for therapists, no how-to books, or seven steps of what to tell clients when you develop a life-threatening disease. Thus, I practiced how to tell them, how much to tell them, and listed their options.

I reframed my having breast cancer as an opportunity for my clients and myself to grow through the process. However, I clearly wanted my clients to feel free to choose what felt best to them. They could stay and continue their work with me, or they could be referred. Some of my clients had already had their appointments changed to accommodate the many tests and doctors' appointments I had carved into my practice schedule. But how much information did they need to know? What would they need from me to cope with the information? How could I help some of them find other therapists?

Pam and I discussed my need to keep my life as normal as possible and not give this disease the benefit of totally rearranging my life. I planned to work through my treatment, at least as much as I was able. I thought it could be a bit unethical to schedule new clients during my treatment, but I believed my current clients needed to be given a choice as whether to stay or seek a referral. This early in the game I had no idea what to expect about how I would do with all of the chemotherapy. However, I did have an idea about how I would feel if my therapist was diagnosed with a life-threatening disease.

I wondered how little information I could actually provide without my clients asking questions. I pride myself on being open, relational, and experiential in my therapeutic demeanor and approach. Honesty and integrity are important to me.

I perused the appointment book and took a look at the names. (All clients' names are fictional, and the personal stories are created. No actual case information is disclosed.)

Sarah, Jason, Suzanne, Denise, Deborah, and Casey – their stories flashed through my head. Several of them were victims of childhood trauma, both sexual and physical abuse. Sarah was the newest client. Her mother had died when Sarah was nine. She ended up living with a grandmother who was mean and demanding. This would not be good news to her. I imagined that she would want a referral. My situation would seem like a nightmare to her. I was thankful that she had only been coming in to see me for a few weeks.

Deborah and Suzanne were friends who were referred by a former client. They would probably stay on, but I wondered how the information would influence them. They both had such trouble developing close connections and I believed Suzanne really suffered from abandonment depression, a chronic depression that keeps good energy blocked in fear of loss. Abandonment threats usually cause this type of client to resolve unconsciously to just "get through this life." Procrastination and apathy dog them.

On the other hand, Deborah had to be broadsided to emit an emotion.

Thus, I expected that she would intellectualize and rationalize the whole experience, and do her darnedest not to feel a thing. I was already very careful with her, not challenging her too much, lest she become really afraid and run. She often had that "deer in the headlights" look on her face when I pushed for her to get in touch with an underlying feeling.

Todd had just come back for a "tune-up" over his relationship. Jason had been here for several years and was still in the same cycle of confusion, trying to decide whether or not to stay married. I worried about him just giving up and going away, either claiming that therapy was a bunch of bull or because of self-blaming beliefs that told him, "You are just not capable of making a choice."

Thomas was finishing up and only coming in on an "as-needed" basis. He was trying to figure out his new relationship.

Then there were Darla, KC, and Erica. They had been coming in for a couple of years now, all three doing intense post-traumatic stress work. Those three would probably be hit hardest with the news because each of them had developed a positive attachment relationship with me. The thought of losing me would be real to them.

I thought I could probably get by without telling some of my clients, at least until I knew whether I was going to lose my hair or not. But if I didn't let these three know directly from me, I knew they would feel very betrayed when they discovered the news. So, how was I really going to do this? I didn't want my information to take up the whole session. I wanted my clients to work as usual throughout their sessions, and then I would break the news during the last fifteen minutes.

I rehearsed, "Darla, I want to wrap up the session a bit early today as I have some information I need to share with you."

"What's that?"

"When I went for this year's mammogram, they found a malignant tumor. I am having a mastectomy next Monday. I will be out of the office for a couple of days, but will be back here on Thursday. I know I will be having chemotherapy afterward, but at this time that's all I know. My plan is to work throughout treatment as much as possible. I have given this much thought and I have created a referral list for you. I want you to continue to obtain the best psychotherapy out there, and to feel free to make the switch to a different therapist. I do not know what I would do if our positions were reversed, but I want you to think about yourself and what you need. The decision to stay or accept a referral has to be yours. I wanted to let you know today so that you have some time to consider what your needs are and what might feel safest to you."

I thought about what I had scripted and tried to put myself in my clients' shoes. If it were my therapist telling me she had breast cancer, what would I want to hear? "Robin, as your therapist who has been working with you over the past few years, I need to let you know I have come up against a bump in my own road. At my last mammogram they discovered a malignant tumor. I am going to have a mastectomy soon."

How would I want to respond to this news? "Yikes, my therapist has breast cancer. What does that mean for me? As for her, will she live?"

Checking in with myself in this way let me know that it felt okay to give my clients as much information as necessary in one short verbal paragraph. It was also helpful to realize that they needed time and permission not to have to respond. Waiting for the last ten to fifteen minutes of the sessions seemed right. They wouldn't be able to think about anything else if I told them at the beginning. If I got them rescheduled soon, they all had enough tools to find ways to deal with the information. It was a usual part of their therapy to journal after their sessions about what emotions and insights they brought away from their session. Also by this time in their therapy they knew how to find a safe place within themselves, how to have internal dialogues, and how to use nature and ritual as ways to help them cope and come to some resolution for themselves.

I feel it is important to teach basic coping and self –soothing skills in the very beginning of the therapeutic relationship. In the following session we could discuss the pros and cons of continuing with me or finding a new therapist.

I ran and reran the rehearsed conversation through my head: "Darla, Erica, K.C., etc., I want to wrap up the session a bit early today as I have some information I need to share with you."

As I ran through the rehearsal one more time in my mind, Darla's story continued to play in my head. I saw scenes from sessions past, where she huddled in a corner and was barely audible as she whispered what it was like to be five years old and have her drunken stepfather come into her room. She told me, "I just wanted my momma. I wanted her to come and make him stop. He stinks and it hurts when he pinches my nipples, and pokes his finger up me. Then I gagged when he forced my head on his penis. Where was my momma?"

She said that the next morning her stepfather told her to be a good little girl and obey her mamma. Don't be bad or I will have to punish you. As she told me this she sobbed, huddled in her little corner. "It was my fault. I was bad."

We spent endless hours going over story after story of trauma, from the age of five, her earliest memory, until she was fourteen. At the age of fourteen her mother caught her stepfather with her, and blamed Darla for seducing the stepfather. She was sent away to live with an aunt in Wyoming. There she was treated like a whore and began her long road down the highway of illicit drugs, permissive sex, and her own battle with alcohol. By the time she was twenty, she was living with an abusive husband and had three small children.   Now at the age of forty-eight, she had raised her children, obtained a B.A. degree, managed an ad agency, and was haunted at nights by recurring dreams of her past. By now she was single, living alone, and shut out anyone who tried to get close to her.

It took Darla about eight months before she really settled in to do any intense work. That is really not unusual for clients with severe trauma histories. She needed to make sure that, regardless of what stories she told me, I wouldn't think she was bad. I prayed a special prayer and asked God for the wisdom in disclosing this news and guidance as to how to say what I needed to say.

I carefully charted the territory of telling each client over the next few days. Each client took the time he or she needed to process the information and express his or her fears. Some clients cried and some became very angry. It gave me the opportunity to see how much my life and my practice of psychotherapy affected each of their lives. It also gave me an opportunity to help them realize that if the outcome was less than we desired their lives would go on and they would find equally experienced therapists to facilitate their psychotherapy journey. The breast cancer taught us that no one is immune to cancer, regardless of his or her life's situation. All clients except one decided to continue their psychotherapy throughout my breast cancer treatment. One client felt it would be too much for her, but neither did she want a referral. She chose to take a hiatus from psychotherapy during my treatment.

My year of active treatment passed and we all made it through, and a month after my hysterectomy I opened my practice to new clients again. I believe the experience of coping with a life-threatening illness has made me a better psychotherapist.

CHAPTER 6

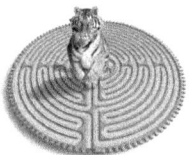

EARLY IMAGES OF CANCER

As I reflected on and struggled with what, when, and how to let my clients know about my cancer, I was thrown back into my history and wondered what part of it made me so personally negative about the disease. I realized I was, indeed, fatalistic about cancer and had been until a client of mine in my Whidbey Island practice taught me that not everyone who gets cancer dies of cancer. I learned a great deal about cancer, life, and the healing power of visualization work through my client, Virginia. Later in this book, you will find a whole chapter dedicated to Virginia.

How did I adopt the belief that everyone who gets cancer dies of cancer? I don't remember any of my family members dying of cancer. My grandmother's death was somewhat of a mystery to me, but I checked that out with my sister, who told me that Grandmother died of congestive heart failure.

Then I remembered. My first real traumatic event occurred the summer when I was four years old. Both my mother and father were blue-collar workers employed at local mills. From the time I was six weeks old, I was cared for daily by Matt – a huge black woman who I loved. I spent more of my waking hours with Matt than I did with my parents. She was there when I woke up in the morning; she took care of me all day, bathed me, changed my diapers, sang to me, and even read to me. It didn't occur to me until I was much older that Matt may not have known how to read. But she certainly told great stories as she pointed to pictures in the books we spent endless hours "reading" together.

As I write this remembering Matt, I smile as Matt's unique body odor drifts through, permeating my olfactory senses, creating a wave of emotions flooding my body with that distinct sensation of being loved. It is easy to recall the feeling of safety and delight as I used to cuddle up in her massive black arms. When I became old enough to talk and to recognize the difference between my white skin and hers of blackest ebony, I asked her, "Why are your hands black, and mine white?"

She told me it was like milk – some milk is white and some milk is chocolate. I said, "I like chocolate best."

We laughed and she fixed me a sipper cup of Nestlé's Quik. I believed for the longest time that chocolate milk came from black cows and white milk came from black and white cows.

Matt adored me and I adored her. We were mirror images of each other – smiling, playing, laughing, and doing what a child and a caregiver do during those long hours before Momma and Daddy come home.

But in my quest for resolution to this bothersome question as to why I believed everyone who got cancer died of cancer, I remembered the pain that later led me to my own therapy and eventual healing. When I was four, going on five, Matt's sister became sick. Matt's sister lived in Ohio. I lived in Virginia. Matt had to leave to take care of her sister and her sister's children. And she never came back. Matt's sister had cancer. Cancer, I understood from the way it was said in such a "hush-hush" manner, was a very bad thing. I came to understand in my young, tender self that cancer takes away those you love and that love you. This early belief was the root of why I think cancer kills anyone it touches. At four, a part of me died when Matt left.

CHAPTER 7

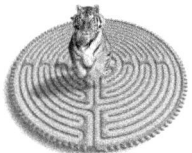

THE MASTECTOMY

At 10:00 a.m. on Monday, August 24, 1999, Dr. BW removed my right breast. As a courtesy to breast cancer patients, insurance companies give a complimentary pass for a one-night hospital stay. My last stay in a hospital had been during a bout with pneumonia at age 16. At that time, I spent the week. My most vivid memory from that experience was the chilling screams from some dark hallway in the hospital during the middle of the night. A nurse told me, "It's nothing to be afraid of, honey. It is just a woman giving birth to a beautiful baby."

Then this nurse brought me an order of french fries from our local Green Mill restaurant. They had the best fries. They were crinkle cuts and the Green Mill would place them in a brown paper bag for take-out. By the time the fries arrived home, all of their grease would discolor the brown bag of fries. I know the nurse intended the french fries to be comfort food. The savory tastes of potato, salt, and grease were extremely satisfying, though they did not drown out the screams from the hallway outside of my room. Besides being comforted, I was aware the french fries carried an unspoken message, a silent bribe requesting that I be a good southern girl child by being quiet and self-contained in my fear.

I don't remember anything about the actual mastectomy surgery. My memory starts with waking up in the recovery room to the words, "You made it," from my comforting partner.

I instinctively reached for my right breast. My fingers recognized the touch of gauze, and I felt relief that I did not have to look at it right away. In my bravery, I was able to look at the tightly wrapped gauze binding the wound from Dr. BW's knife.

The nurses checked on me. One nurse, Janet, was particularly informative and comforting. She had undergone a mastectomy just three years before. She told a funny story: "My husband, son, and I went to the beach last summer. When I was getting out of the ocean and returning for my beach towel, I noticed I was missing my prosthesis. I yelled to my son, 'Quick, start looking for my boob. It's missing.' My son and my husband got up and began to walk along the shoreline when my son noticed a small floating object about three waves out. He yelled, 'Hey, mom, I think that's your boob.' He swam out and rescued it. It was rather soggy and limp, but after getting the salt water out, it was just like new." Janet finished her story by telling me that, "Having a mastectomy becomes a family thing." That was something I was learning.

I noticed the tubes creeping out of the gauze. I fingered them carefully and followed them to the end where there were two round plastic bulbs. The bulbs collected the blood and amber-colored fluid draining from my wound. As I asked questions about these bulbs, Janet instructed me about how I would drain and measure the fluid on a daily basis and told me exactly how many ounces I would be collecting. "Each day the fluid will decrease in amount and when it gets to one cubic centimeter, then Dr. BW will remove them," she told me.

The fluid made me nauseated. I didn't stare at it very long. It was hard to imagine such ugly looking stuff coming out of my body.

Janet brought me a Popsicle. I listened to the conversations around me. It became increasingly clear that the hospital did not have a patient room for me. The clock on the wall showed 4:00 p.m. I just wanted to sleep. There was still no evidence of a room. Pam and I had no privacy to share any of the intimacies that we desired to share with each other after such a horrible ordeal. We stared at each other in tenderness, and beneath the tenderness our souls shared a deep fear.

Nurses kept coming by and, with artificial cheerfulness that even a child would not believe, said "Soon! They are clearing you a room right now."

I was too tired to fight. What good would it do? If they didn't have a room, they didn't have a room. My sarcastic imagination ran away, creating a funny image from the nurse's statement, "We are clearing a room for you now."

I imagined an old crotchety nurse named Bertha holding a pillow over a patient's head until the life is completely snuffed out and saying, "Sorry, your time has expired. I need this room for another patient." I reminded myself that I had better not ask too many questions if I am going to be Nurse Bertha's next patient.

Finally, just as dark was settling in, a team of nurses came and rolled me on a gurney to a room three flights up. I was lifted into a bed, and Pam and I had some alone time at last. I remember thinking, *Finally, I can hold her hand and she mine while we say nothing and hope for the best.*

Pam was exhausted, too. This was a devastating ride for both of us. Indeed a mastectomy is a family thing.

I hated that she had to go home by herself. I so wanted the comfort of my own home, our bed, and our dog, Bobbin, and cat, Schnapps. However, it didn't take long for sleep to overcome me. Pam kissed me, and then told me "I will see you in the morning."

A nurse appeared, took my temperature and blood pressure, and then I withdrew into my most inner self to contemplate what my life would be like next. I touched my gauze one last time with the same caution and tenderness that I had used the night before when I held my right breast in the palm of my hand, bent my head down and kissed it, saying good-bye to it as tears flowed down my checks. Now in some strange way I was holding the gauze that protected my wound, attempting to say good-bye and hello at the same time.

There is an old world story, the "Miller's Daughter," that has a line in it at one of the most important junctures for the girl in the story – a line that punctuates the change taking place: "Life as she knew it came to an end."

That was exactly what was happening to Pam and me as we attempted to embrace this travesty and make the most of it.

CHAPTER 8

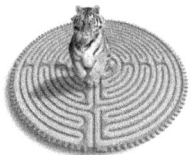

THE NEXT FEW DAYS

The white bandage across my chest with tubes nudging out of tight crevices was there to greet me the next morning, along with another strange nurse wanting to check my vitals. After she left, I touched the bandage, still relieved that I did not have to look beneath to what I imagined to be a gaping hole turning into a very ugly scar. I falsely imagined the scar would be a circle. However, I knew that it would be linear in nature going from under my armpit across my chest. I just wasn't ready to face the reality that my body was now permanently altered. The permanence of it all had yet to sink in. I was just not able to acknowledge the harsh reality of it yet.

The decision to complete the mastectomy without reconstruction is now a permanent part of my life. It is true that it is important to me that based on current insurance rules I am still entitled to undergo breast reconstruction if I should ever choose to do so. Actually, the law uses the word "symmetrical." Perhaps in the future I will choose surgery to create symmetry and have the remaining breast removed. However, I imagine that if I ever decide to do anything that one day I might get a tattoo across my chest. Deena Metzger, the author of *Writing for Your Life*, is reported to have a tree tattooed where her breast used to be. Maybe one day, I will have a tattoo artist draw a powerful tiger guarding over me from where my right breast used to be.

I knew that when I looked at my scar the first time I wanted to be in a private place, a place where I alone could touch, caress, cry or swear. I just wanted that moment for the first time between my scar and me to be a private one.

I distracted myself by wondering where in the geographical context of the world my right breast had gone. A part of my body was missing and I had no idea where it was. Was it wrapped in some cold solution, floating in a plastic bag in the back of a UPS truck, traveling to some obscure sterile lab? Once they dissected my breast and finalized their pathology report, would they just toss the rest of the tissue in a trash can and dump it in the dumpster? My rational self said, "No, they toss it in a hospital incinerator and reduce it to non-diseased ash."

I never really asked anyone. I left myself with the above assumption; it was an assumption with which I could live. A wave of sadness overcame me, but quickly abated when the words "Good morning, my love" danced into my room. Pam with her beautiful smile had arrived.

We touched the bandage, looked at the now-full bulbs of fluid, and inspected the worry in each other's eyes as we wondered silently what would come next. The immediate next was proving I could walk and go to the bathroom so that the hospital could dutifully kick me out at noon. I demonstrated that I could do both. "Since I have passed your test, I want to go home now," I requested.

No doctor visit was required. However I did fantasize telling the nursing staff, "Please be sure to thank the insurance company for my complimentary stay and tell them not to take it personally that I wanted to leave at 8:00 a.m. I just want to go home."

Safe at home, I turned to the TV to help escape the horror. I walked around the house in a daze. I wanted to wake up from the nightmare and get back to how life used to be. Pam's 49th birthday came and went without any real hoopla. I felt bad about that.

Finally, it was time for the bandage to be changed. I knew I would have to face my scar. Gently I took the gauze and tape off, layer by layer.

There the scar lay beneath the white gauze, red and swollen, tender to the touch, and ugly. I gently touched it, caressed it, and looked at it in the mirror. I felt very sad. Pulling quickly away from a barrage of emotion, I said, "Okay, baby. It is you and me now. Welcome to my life." I placed the bandages on it and turned my attention to some chore that lay unfinished to distract me from the sadness.

In just a few short days, my life had changed forever. The fluid tubes around my neck were in the way. They pulled on my neck. They were bothersome and ugly, and smelly fluid just kept filling them up. Sitting down at the dinner table was an awkward experience. The bulbs would then lie in my lap, peeping out beneath my shirt. It was not very appetizing to eat and realize that my body fluids were hanging around in full view. I was not scheduled to see Dr. BW until the following week. It would take about seven days for the fluid to drain, and then he would go over the results with me and remove the tubes at the same time.

CHAPTER 9

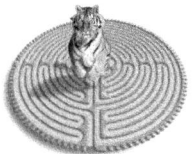

THE FIRST TEARS

Again, I knew without being told that the cancer was in my lymph nodes. I just knew. It was after the mastectomy that my denial wore very thin. I had the discomfort of the mastectomy, the reality of the scar, and the real intrusions into my daily life with doctor appointments and trips to medical centers for other tests. I was becoming tired and irritable with it all. As Pam and I walked up the steps to Dr. BW's office on that hot day near the end of August, I felt the tension and that ominous feeling of anxiety like a coiled rattlesnake, prepared to strike. My warrior-self was on notice. My environmental senses were heightened. My normal state of being had become one of hyper-arousal. Hyper-arousal is a symptom of Post Traumatic Stress Disorder, and my PTSD was quickly taking over my state of consciousness.

As Dr. BW entered the examination office, all pleasantries were bypassed. There was the brief question, "How much liquid are you collecting and what color is it?" he asked.

I replied, "There is very little liquid and it is now only the color of straw – no blood is still draining."

It was almost like I hadn't said a word. His mind was clearly somewhere else, other than on the amount of straw-colored liquid in these bulbs dangling from my neck. Before I could process the obvious tension between us, he pulled out the pathology report with this introduction, "I am surprised by your pathology report. Your cancer has invaded eight of twelve lymph nodes."

There was nothing like those words, "I am surprised."

My eyes automatically, without permission, filled with a deluge of scorching hot tears. My chest silently heaved, refusing to let another sliver of breath in or out. I sat there exposed in that silly office gown. I had no safe words, no words that were socially acceptable. The more I tried not to cry, the more my chin quivered and the blotchier the red spots around my mouth became.

Telling a patient, "You have cancer," must be the hardest part of a doctor's job. And even though she or he probably tells someone that every day – "I am sorry, you have cancer" – there is just no easy or right way to do it. Dr. BW handed me a tissue and spoke the truth. "I know this was not what you wanted to hear."

He was right. I did not want to hear those words. Those words broke through any denial I had left within me. I had known all along that it had traveled to my lymph nodes. I just wanted to be wrong. I could find no breath to help me communicate anything to him. I went into computer mode the best I could and asked a couple of questions and we all managed to refocus on the pathology report. He brought to my attention a very important part of the report by pointing out to me that the pathology reported detected another tumor, 3.5. cm in size, hidden deep with my breast tissue as well as discovering other infiltrating microscopic foci.

All of these words meant one thing: they had found another tumor even bigger than the bump. This undetected tumor was hiding deep within the dense breast tissue so it did not show up on the mammogram or the ultrasound. If I had not had the mastectomy that tumor would have remained concealed deep in the breast tissue.

My final diagnosis was Stage Two Aggressive Estrogen Positive Ductal

Carcinoma. I knew then that chemotherapy would not be at my discretion. I was still trying to hold on to those tears as Dr. BW finished the report. I desperately wanted to banish the tears to that secret place inside of me but, regardless of how hard I tried, they bubbled over the top. Dr. BW handed me another tissue and Pam just looked so heartbroken.

There were times during this journey when I thought, *No, I can't do this. Just let me die now.* This was one of those times. The denial now was gone, shattered from its eclipse of his words "because of the tumor's small size, we do not expect it has traveled to the lymph nodes."
However, there was a tad bit of emotional relief about finding the other tumor, as its discovery validated that I had made the right decision to have the mastectomy.

I did not have time to continue to process those feelings as Dr. BW continued, "You're right, the drainage is coming along. I can go ahead and remove those tubes. It will sting a bit."

Yes, in fact, it did sting, but what was more surprising was how much tubing was inside of my body. Well over a yard of plastic tubing just kept coming out of the hole under my arm. I guess there is no neat way to get those tubes out. In a matter of fact voice, Pam commented afterward, "I don't even think he had gloves on and the fluid just dripped everywhere."

He tossed the tubing into the trash can and then we discussed my options for quite a while. I had already chosen an oncologist so this report would be sent to him. During the rest of the discussion, I could not stop focusing on the non-detected tumor.

I asked again, "How big was it? How could it not show up? I thought the mammogram would detect it."

Dr. BW explained, "It is tumors just like that one that I believe cause the recurrence in patients who choose only lumpectomies. However, what your oncologist and radiologist will probably tell you is that even if a tumor is not discovered, the radiation and chemotherapy should take care of it."

I know I was quite distressed when he was talking, but I can remember saying to myself in my satirical sort of way, "Oh well, if chemotherapy and radiation are so powerful, why have a mastectomy in the first place? Just let those procedures take care of everything after the biopsy."

I have always had a difficult time with the "god-like" presence of the medical profession and now I was sure my entry into the depths of it would be extremely taxing. I found their logic to be self-serving at times. In the past, I often heard reports of male surgeons trying to talk women into lumpectomies to save their breasts. Every time I heard a report of this nature I became indignant. I am thankful I didn't have to work with a surgeon who thought my breasts were more important than my life. I was also very appreciative that Dr. BW was very forthcoming with the statistics of recurrence in lumpectomies versus mastectomies. I think finding that second undetected tumor made me more anxious than the fact the cancer had spread to the lymph nodes. There was just something unsettling about discovering that a villain was living secretly in my body.

That sense that a secret intruder has invaded my body is still a feeling that I try to deal with emotionally. How does that happen without me knowing it is there? There are many unfair and scary things about breast cancer, or any cancer, but the reality that it can grow and take over my body unbeknownst to me is just bone chilling. The secrecy created a feeling that my body was somehow against me. I felt my body had betrayed me and felt as if I was stalked by some stranger inside of my own body. Those are some of the dark feelings that I still grapple with today as I try to make sense out of this journey.

I don't remember anything else about that day. I know I just wanted to go to that secret place deep inside of myself and stay there. My mother has been dead since 1993, but at times like this I still fought hard not to want her. I just wanted to run home to Mom, hoping she would kiss the "owie" and make it go away. I know deep inside though that, even if she had still been alive, I wouldn't have wanted to worry her.

My appointment with my oncologist was not until September 3rd.

Pam and I returned to our cabin in Happy Jack for Labor Day. We poured over *Susan Love's Breast Health Book*. When I went for my first appointment with my oncologist, I was loaded with intelligent questions from the book: What is in the biopsy report that actually determines that this is an aggressive cancer? What types of chemotherapy drugs will you be using? Why are you making those choices? How soon can we start the treatment? Statistically what are my numbers for survival with this type of cancer?

I received the answers to those questions even though I was suffering from severe oxygen deprivation due to shallow breathing (better known in my field as "anxiety") during that visit.

CHAPTER 10

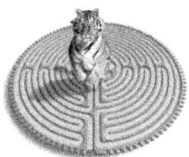

OXYGEN DEPRIVATION AND DISTORTED REALITY

I love my oncologist. Dr. Martin Langford showed me respect throughout my treatment. He seemed to appreciate and value my participation in my recovery all the way through my six months of treatment and the ten years of ongoing follow-up. We got off to a hilarious start – a start that I am sure he is unaware of and that I hope he will find amusing if he ever decides to read this book.

In the oncology waiting room, Pam and I masked our shock as we silently noted the patients – young, old, male, female – all frail and hairless. I noticed Pam watching a baby less than two years old. I knew children got leukemia but I guess I thought all children received treatment at a children's hospital, locked away someplace where I was protected from seeing their hollow eyes and tender faces. Children are just too young to go through this. But the child, a toddler, was walking back and forth between two adults.

At first, I tried to make one of the two adults the cancer patient. But my eyes could not escape the dreadfulness of such young sunken eyes and a diminished body. Both adults appeared healthy and I quickly projected my worry for the child onto them. How horrible for a baby that is cherished, wanted, and loved to have to battle for her little life. *How are these caregivers coping? How did they discover the cancer? What type of cancer is it? Will she live? What does her little soul make out of those needles and tubes pushing their way into her little body? What does she think? What does she know? What is she able to comprehend?*

The bombardment of internal questions was interrupted when the nurse appeared and called the name of the child. I watched the adults take her by the hands and she toddled unafraid through the door to the nurse. I was flooded with emotion. Pam's eyes watered. I quickly grabbed a magazine – it didn't matter which one. There was no chance that I would actually read it, but I certainly was going to do my damnedest to pretend to read as my eyes continually scanned the periphery of the room.

I observed the obvious wigs, colorful scarves and hats, and some brave bald heads. I knew I would choose to be boldly bald. I hate any type of hat or scarf. To my amusement and horror, in the middle of the waiting room amidst this entire travesty of people dealing with life and death issues, a chemotherapy patient marked by her colorful bandanna was eating a McDonald's lunch. I wanted to throw-up. *How could someone eat among so much destruction? Couldn't other people see what I saw? This was a place of death. Where were the mourners and hired wailers?*

Everyone seemed to be trying to normalize this experience as if we were all there to be treated for the common cold. The emotional shock of it all sent me reeling. But on the outside, I appeared cool and calm, just like everyone else in the waiting room. It was just another day, just another doctor's visit. Somewhere after my tears in Dr. BW's office, I had regrouped and re-entered that deep dark place inside of me where no one could read my reactions.

Finally the nurse called, "Robin Dilley." Of course, this was before HIPAA and the federal government's inept attempt at privacy, so attendants still used both first and last names. Now, under the new HIPAA privacy act, the attending nurse calls only the first name, so when John or Bob is in a medical waiting room, all six of them look up at the same time, wondering who the nurse really wants.

A smile, a curious "how are you today?" greeted Pam and me as we crossed the threshold from one medical nightmare to a different one. From the hall I could see the other patients in the actual chemotherapy room. However, the routine was familiar - I weighed in just like all of the other doctors' offices I have ever been in. Then, our escort took us to one of those doctors' chambers where I saw the standard jar of cottons balls, tissue box, and a poster of the human body on the wall. A different nurse entered and took my vitals, my temperature, blood pressure, and pulse.

Less than a week earlier at Dr. BW's office, I was told to never again allow my blood pressure to be taken or my blood to be drawn from my mastectomy side, which is my right. Someone also told me not to ever wear fingernail polish again, and to wear gloves when digging in the dirt. I hate gloves as much as I do hats, so I don't do so well on that one, but it was a long time after treatment before I painted my nails again. The chemicals in the nail polish are hard on the lymph system, and I believed taking these small precautions helped me protect my compromised lymph node system.

The nurse finished taking my vitals and said, "Take off your top and put on the gown opening to the front. The doctor will be in shortly."

The nurse closed the door behind her and I did what I was instructed. Soon a very young-looking doctor walked in with his clipboard and my pathology report. He immediately addressed me as "Dr. Dilley." I appreciated the formality and his willingness to recognize my accomplishments.

He pulled up the round doctor's stool and sat, propping his head up with his elbow resting on the counter. I sat on the edge of the examination table, and Pam was in the chair to my left. I introduced her and he warmly greeted her and extended his hand.

"I know this has been a rough ride for both of you," he said. "And quite frankly, Dr. Dilley, I am very surprised by your pathology report. Your tumor was less than 1.2 mm. Under most circumstances, it doesn't travel to the lymph node system until it is larger. So this is an aggressive type."

I said nothing, but noticed a tickle beginning deep in my belly. I wanted to laugh.

He continued, "We will give you eight rounds of chemotherapy. The first four rounds will be a mixture of Adriamycin and Cytoxan. The last four treatments will be with a newer drug, Taxol. Taxol is a plant derivative and we are experiencing quite a bit of success with its use."

"Success with, success with, s...ucce...sss w...i...th"– the words sounded funny. They rolled around in my head and off of my tongue like they were billiard balls split by the cue a thousand times over.

I finally reached what seemed to be a perfectly logical conclusion. This guy's voice was funny. He sounded just like Donald Duck.

I looked at him. He didn't have a duck bill, or webbed feet. But his cadence and tone of voice was that of Donald Duck.

I wondered, *How in the world did anyone take him seriously in medical school? How many patients he has seen? Does anyone ever laugh in his face?*

I drifted back to his monologue. "Your cancer is aggressive; it is stage two estrogen positive. As a result, you may want to consider a study they are doing at a local research center. The study is for stage two breast cancer patients. Basically what they are doing is using very aggressive doses of chemotherapy drugs after they extract your bone marrow. They call that harvesting and then they replace your bone marrow after treatment. I will be happy to make you a referral."

Dr. Donald Duck continued, "If you opt for the study, you will receive all of your treatments at the research center and there will be no reason for you to come back here."

I replied, "Go ahead and arrange an appointment for me down there and I will check it out. You say it is called a stem cell transplant?"

"Yes. I'll have Cody make you an appointment. Go ahead and schedule here for no later than the 13th. You can cancel this appointment if you decide to enter the study; otherwise, I do not want to waste any time getting the chemotherapy started."

What this good doctor could not tell by my lack of facial expression was that I was ready to burst out laughing. *If he doesn't shut up I am going to laugh in his face*, I thought. Here was this educated man talking to me about all of this scientific stuff and somehow he had a voice anomaly that made him sound just like Donald Duck.

"Also, Dr. Dilley, we need to see exactly how far the cancer has spread, so we will need to have a chest x-ray, a CT scan, a bone scan and some blood work. We will go ahead and schedule those for you, too. Even if you decide to do the study, they will need all of those tests."

Cancer spread. I repeated those words to myself. I thought we already knew it was in eight out of twelve lymph nodes. What did he mean, "*spread?*"

I didn't ask because I was afraid if I used my voice to say any more I might start laughing and not be able to stop. I offered a blank and mute stare. On that note, he stood up, shook our hands again and said, "It is nice to meet you both and I look forward to hearing from you. Good day."

The door closed behind him. I just wanted out of his office. As I started putting my shirt back on, I burst into laughter.

"What's so funny?" Pam asked.

"I'll tell you when we get out of here."
After I was fully dressed, we left, met Cody – a cute and personable assistant – and she scheduled me for the blood work, bone scan, CT scan, and chest x-ray and at the research center all within a few minutes. I moved to the next counter to pay my co-pay and I inquired, "How long has Dr. F been in practice?"

The receptionist said, "Oh, for a long time, but he just moved here from a practice in New York."

"Oh really, he looks very young," I replied.

She looked at me as if to check from which planet I had arrived. She looked around and said, "There is Dr. F right there."

The man she pointed to was an older, heavier, and balder person than the one who had entered my examining room.

"Hmm," I said in a somewhat distressed tone. "That's not who I saw. The doctor I saw was much younger. My appointment was supposed to be with F. I saw the wrong doctor."

What I didn't say was, "he talks like a duck."

She looked at me and smiled. "No, you saw Dr. Langford. He is one of the original doctors here. We changed you to Dr. Langford because he's on your insurance plan and Dr. F is not."

"Oh," I said. "No one told me."

I signed my name to the twenty-five dollar check for my co-pay and got lost in the attempt to exit without glancing to my right where all of the baldheaded skinny, frail patients were sitting. Pam and I found our way out to the parking lot where I could not stop laughing. She, of course, wanted to know why, and I said, "Didn't you think that doctor sounded just like Donald Duck?"

She looked at me, very puzzled, and said, "No, that's not how he sounded to me."

She was serious. I was confused. "He certainly sounded just like Donald Duck."

I laughed it off until the next visit. During my second visit I listened keenly for Donald Duck, but he was nowhere to be found. Stress leads to oxygen deprivation, which leads to brain dysfunction, often including hallucinations, delusions, or just plain old misperceptions.

My admiration for Dr. Langford is still present after our years of working together. He has never let me down. Three years after my surgery, I turned the corner of a corridor in a hospital. In my role as a psychologist, I was visiting a patient who was battling pancreatic cancer. There I saw my oncologist sitting at the nurse's station, charting in a patient's file. A bubble of mutual respect spilled its warmth over us. I went to him and said, "Hello."

His broad smile welcomed me. "What brings you to this side of town?"

"I'm seeing one of my favorite patients who is struggling to recover from invasive pancreatic cancer surgery. She just turned eighty in January."

"I didn't know you came all the way over here. I had you in the Thunderbird area," he said.

"No, I have always had Scottsdale clients. Now with the new freeway, the 101, just makes our lives easier. I thought about having a satellite office over here, but with the 101 that is hardly necessary," I said. "Are you going to be my client's oncologist?"

"Who is her doctor?" he asked.

"Dr. Short."

"Probably not. Her doctor uses a different oncology team."

"That's too bad," I said. "They don't know what they are missing."

He asked, "How are you doing?"

"Hey, I am good to go. That PET scan we did in December didn't come up with anything."

"I see you in a couple of months, don't I?" he asked.

"This summer, I think," I said.

It was not until my drive away from the hospital that I realized he wanted to do a four-month check because of my continual battle with crazy blood work. I also reflected on Clara, my pancreatic cancer patient. I felt sad as I thought about her, full of life, vim, vigor, and goals she still wanted to meet. At eighty she still had amazing plans for herself. Even after her unfortunate fall which resulted in a broken hip last autumn, she had fully recovered. She was looking forward to going to the Cape for the summer and enjoying Arizona's perfect spring. But by February, she was diagnosed with pancreatic cancer, and by April her medical team talked this poor lady into Whipple surgery. That surgery is an invasive, drastic, and a completely insane thing to do to an eighty-year-old who is going to die of cancer. However, I don't get to make medical decisions for my clients, which is a good thing. Making my own decisions is hard enough.

Cancer has its own particular way of becoming real, again and again and again. I can go for a period of time and then not even think about it except during my healing ritual. But then in the middle of doing my job, here it comes all over again.

CHAPTER 11

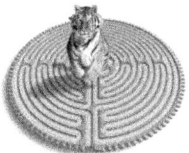

STEM CELL TRANSPLANT

Shortly after my first visit with Dr. Langford, oxygen deprivation occurred again during my interview for a stem cell transplant. Actually it is entirely possible that my level of trauma superseded anxiety and became more like the symptoms of physical shock. Stem cells – or auto transplants as they are often referred to – are lifesavers for some patients. If I had been diagnosed with stage three or stage four breast cancer, then I may have made a different decision. However, in 1999, the research on stem cell transplants showed that there was only slight statistical significance between a stem cell transplant and the standard of care for stage two breast cancer.

I must have downloaded a full ream of paper with all of the then-current information on stem cell transplants and breast cancer studies. Unfortunately, I did not save the reams to give you the sites I found. But I did locate one 1999 study that provides a great description of stem cell transplants and the statistics at that time. That newspaper article stated, "Three-year survival rate was not statistically significant among 184 women who got transplants vs. standard chemotherapy for metastatic breast cancer in a study by the Eastern Cooperative Oncology group, a coalition of American Cancer Centers."

It went on to state that a small study in France of 61 participants and a Scandinavian study of 525 women found no statistical significance. That article also provided me with a study of 873 high risk breast cancer patients that didn't fare any better over a five-year period of time versus those who received the standard of care for stages three and four breast cancer. The total data in this article stated that in 1999 only 1,000 women were in clinical trials for stem cell transplants but 16,000 women had obtained the transplant without being part of a study. Thus, that group of 16,000 does not count in the data collection of successes or failures of stem cell transplants. The cost for a transplant in 1999 would have been $60,000 to $70,000.

When Pam and I found the words "stem cell transplant" we more often than not found the words "bone marrow" transplant adjacent to them. There is a difference between stem cell and bone marrow transplants but my understanding is that bone marrow transplants are conducted to treat other types of cancers, such as leukemia. Bone marrow is a spongy material that is found inside of our bones, particularly the pelvic bone. Bone marrow is like a factory and produces red blood cells, white blood cells and platelets. Red blood cells carry oxygen to all cells in our bodies. White blood cells are essential in fighting infection and platelets help blood clot and prevent bleeding. Stem cells are generic precursor cells found in circulating blood. The precursor cells develop into all three types of blood cells: white, red, and platelets. They can be taken from the bone marrow or from the blood stream.

Transplantation involves filtering a patient's blood for several days to remove stem cells and storing those cells under controlled conditions. Next, the patient is given high-dose chemotherapy, which fights the cancer but has the side effect of killing any remaining bone marrow. By transplanting the stem cells back into the body, the body is given the resource it needs to recover from the chemotherapy.

Chemotherapy is poison. It is "good for you" poison because cancerous growing tumors are tenacious and do not give up their hold on your system without a lethal battle. Each year, new revised chemotherapy drugs are researched in order to continue to fight against deadly cancerous diseases. As I said in Chapter One, when I was diagnosed with breast cancer, I thought all breast cancers were alike. I didn't understand the staging of breast cancer other than my own interpretation which was that the higher the stage, the closer the door of death.

I certainly had no understanding of estrogen positive, progesterone positive or HER2 breast cancer. I didn't hear the words "inflammatory breast cancer" until a year after my treatment began. I didn't understand the DNA results on my pathology report nor did I know that various chemotherapy drugs targeted different types of cancers. As late as 2004 the medical field was just gaining a very basic understanding of DNA and how to target it for treatment of cancer.

Stages and Types of Breast Cancer in 2010.

Because I am neither a medical doctor nor a cancer specialist, I am not going to go into detail about the various and diverse types of breast cancers. However, I am providing you with some basics and then you can begin your search on the web or ask your medical doctor for further information. The words on this list you may hear on television or used by family or friends.

There are eight clinical stages of breast cancer, ranging from Stage 0 to Stage IV. In between those numbers are: Stage 0, Stage I, Stage II A, Stage II B, Stage III A, Stage III B, Stage III C and Stage IV.

A simple rule of thumb is the larger the stage, the more aggressive and invasive the cancer.

For instance, Stage 0 means that cancer cells exist and are contained in breast ducts or lobules.   By contrast, Stage IV means that the cancer has spread to other organs in the body, most often the liver, lungs, or brain.

Other terminology that you may hear used often:
- *Ductal Carcinoma in Situ*: 1 in 5 breast cancers; cancer contained in the ductal area of the breast.
- *Invasive Carcinoma*: Most cancers are invasive or often called infiltrating.

- **Hormone Receptors**: Proteins on the breast cancer cells. These receptors pick up signals from the hormones estrogen, progesterone, and HER 2 (Human Growth Factor Receptor 2), enabling the cancer cells to grow.
- **Estrogen Positive or Estrogen Negative**: Simply means that estrogen receptors are present or not present in the breast cancer cells. If estrogen receptors are present, then the estrogen feeds the cancer.
- **Progesterone Positive or Progesterone Negative**: Either progesterone receptors are present or not in the breast cancer cells.
- **HER2**: A gene mutation of a protein called human epidermal growth factor receptor 2 (HER2) which promotes the growth of cancer cells.
- **Triple Negative**: None of the above are present and the cancer cells are more like basal cells. This cancer is more prevalent in younger women under fifty, the African-American and Hispanic populations, and those who have the BRACA I gene mutation (hereditary).
- **Inflammatory (IBC)**: Uncommon invasive breast cancer; accounts for only 1-3% of all breast cancers. Usually there is no tumor, but the breast become red, warm, itchy and often very tender. Often the breast become thick pitted in appearance similar to that of an orange peel.
- **Grade**: At the time I was diagnosed, there were no grades on my pathology report. Today grades consist of 1-3. Again, the larger the grade the less differentiated the cell, adding severity to the diagnosis.

This small glossary is only the beginning of a medical language that you must learn if you or your family member or friend is diagnosed with breast cancer. The stage, the grade, and the type of breast cancer determine how your medical team will recommend treatment.

Because the success rate of a stem cell transplant was not statistically different from the success rate for the standard of care, I was looking at all of the dangers and problems with the studies. I still considered myself young at forty-five. I wanted to live to be old enough to wear purple and to have the best quality of life I could have. I didn't want any of my other organs, such as my liver, heart, or kidneys to be compromised more than necessary. The high doses of chemotherapy would damage all of the other parts of my body and I would be on disability, because I would be too weak to work. I clearly understood from my research that I would be taken to death's door by the mega doses of chemotherapy. Certainly that was a trip I preferred not to take. But I attempted to have an open mind when I went to the orientation session at a local hospital to look further at my options.

CHAPTER12

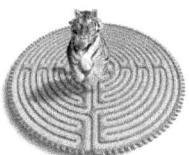

THE STEM CELL ORIENTATION

My appointment with the center was at 2:00 p.m. We arrived on time, but not early, thank goodness. As we entered the research center's doors, it was apparent that we had entered into an entirely different world of medicine. It was big and ominous. The corridors were flocked with patients and white coats. People were coming and going on the many elevator systems.

At the information booth for new patients, the receptionist gave us a map to negotiate the hugeness of this hospital. If I were searching for research patients, I think I would at least attempt to hide the realities about what to expect until the end of the interview.

I saw two things, both at the same time – a former acquaintance, Joe, who I hadn't seen in several years – and the patients behind glass, bald and dressed in pale yellow hospital gowns.

I heard the sound of the machines pumping. Joe was working in the unit and he was in charge of registering me. I felt tears for the second time. Seeing someone I knew and liked while having to deal with this cancer thing brought a lump into my throat.

My eyes rapidly scanned the unit. I couldn't stop my attention from focusing on the windowed room just behind Joe's right shoulder. I concentrated on the sound of the pumping machine rather than looking at the bald heads in yellow gowns. The shock factor was making my heart race as if I had entered a bad episode in the Twilight Zone. The hairless patients looked very old and fragile.

Pam and I were seated in an area within the unit to fill out the paperwork. In my view from that seat was another windowed room with other yellow-robed patients. I believe they were children. However, by this time I had successfully escaped to that place deep inside of myself. I shut off my mind, not allowing in any further information, fearing that I was about to faint. I became completely dissociated, sufficiently watching my experience from the ceiling. I was hidden deep in my internal cave and only a dim light allowed me to see the things I needed to see, like the words on the forms. And once again, just less than a month from diagnosis I was writing "breast cancer" as the reason for treatment or testing. Even today, years later, those words do not roll easily off of my tongue.

As I finished the paperwork, a tall doctor in a dark suit, white shirt, and tie came to escort us down another hall to a conference corner – not even a private room. I didn't particularly like him but that may have been because I was deep into my cave and I didn't want him to "get me." By this time, after viewing all of those patients in yellow gowns, I was not feeling safe. The doctor seemed like a predator to me.

"I have my tape recorder. I would like to tape the session," I said.

Clearly a bit taken aback, he responded, "Sure that will be fine."

"I know there will be lots of information exchanged. I know that within an hour after this appointment I will not be able to remember really important things. I want to hear and rehear my questions and your answers," I said.

The three of us spent about two hours together listening, and asking and answering questions. I knew as I was following the doctor down the long corridor that my mind was clearly made up, but the researcher inside of me still wanted all of the information I could get.

I had one last question for him. Prior to choosing my treatment, I enlisted information from my family doctor, medical friends like my sister-in-law, second opinions, and questioned other medical professionals who were already involved in my journey. I told them, "I am a candidate for a stem cell transplant study. I want to check it out, but I want to go into the interview as prepared as possible. I want to place as many odds in my favor as possible."

I found one particular question to be very helpful to me as I tried to do just that, put all of the odds in my favor. In a discussion with a member of my medical team I was asked, "Robin how many patients are a part of this study? If you decide to participate in this clinical trial then go to the facility where there are there are a lot of patients and the treatment team is well seasoned. It is very important that there is a team approach to the study and that the team knows what they are doing and what to expect."

My final question to this aloof-looking doctor was, "How many participants do you already have in this study?" This study had been open for one year at the time.

The doctor answered, "One. Actually, three patients participated in the stem cell transplant, but only one of them met the actual criteria for the study."

He then went on to remind me that if I chose to pursue this option of treatment that the computer may not choose me for the study. I could however, opt for the treatment; I just would not be a part of the study, meaning my data would not count toward any further information about stem cell transplants. If we go back and look at the 16,000 women who chose a stem cell transplant as their method of treatment, we do not have their data. We only have the data of the 1,000 American women in the study by 1999. What a waste of information. Nonetheless, I had my final answer.

 I told the doctor, "Based on my prior research of this procedure and the information I gathered here today, I am choosing to pass on this option at this time. My odds seem to be just as good with the standard of care and I believe that is the best choice for my body at this time. If I change my mind, I will give you a call in a few days."

We shook hands and Pam and I left. It took several hours to decompress from what had been an overload to my sensory system, and when I go back there in my memory bank, I am still filled with terror.

CHAPTER 13

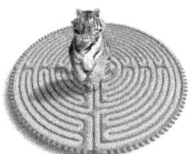

EMBRACING THE TEACHER IN BREAST CANCER

One of the ways that I cope with difficult issues in my life is to view them as teachers. Honoring the situation empowers me to rise above the victim's stance and the accompanying plaintive whine: "Woe is me, isn't my life awful?"

Looking at breast cancer as a metaphorical teacher moves it a step or two outside of me. The operative word here is "metaphor." If I view breast cancer as a teacher, I free myself to enter my relationship with it in a much different way, a way that invites curiosity. The curious position is that as a psychologist I am used to implementing in my practice. I am trained to stay curious, to ask questions.

For instance, when a client such as Sarah says, "I wish that I could just go to sleep tonight and wake up in the morning and this nightmare would be over," I know that Sarah has regressed into a state of mind which mirrors that of a wishful child who still believes in Santa Claus.

Rather than challenging that position, I use a narrative or strategic approach by wondering out loud. "Well, let's play with that a bit. What would be different tomorrow if you went to bed tonight and a miracle happened?"

Sarah says, "Well my boyfriend would be considerate and act as if he cares about me."

"Oh, I see. You want the miracle for him and not for yourself?"

Sarah says, "Yes, if he would just be different then I would be happy."

"Well, Sarah. I'm curious about why it is that you want John to make you happy. You are a bright, intelligent woman. Why do you put John in charge of your happiness?"

"I don't do that," Sarah says adamantly.

"Oh, you just wanted the miracle for John out of the goodness of your heart," I say gently.

Sarah then is able to see how silly it is that she wants John to change to make her happy. She begins to realize that she really must step up to the plate and truly decide whether she wants to stay with someone who never hears her or who doesn't act very interested in her life and dreams.

Breast cancer arrived in my life. I did nothing to invite it in. God did not send it to me. It simply arrived and I choose how to view it. If I view it as an awful thing, if I allow myself to lapse into the role of a victim ("what did I do so wrong that this is happening to me?" or "why me?" said in a martyred voice) then I give breast cancer a position of power over me. I give myself a sense of empowerment by choosing how I viewed its role in my life. By deciding to see breast cancer as a teacher that arrived, then I have the option of personalizing it, asking questions like, "why me?" – but rather than in a blaming tone, from a place inside that asks, "Okay, now that you have arrived, what am I supposed to do with you?"

By seeing breast cancer as my teacher, I allow myself to ask many questions about its role in my life. What is it I am supposed to be learning? What am I not attending to that needs my attention? If a miracle happens tonight how will my life be different tomorrow? What stops me from making that different right now?

Just a few months prior to my being diagnosed with breast cancer, I self-published a personal growth journal in the spring of 1999. That journal, ***Writing Your Way to Healing and Wholeness: Simple Exercises for Exploring Your Past and Creating Your Future*** started off with asking the writer to create three wishes. The rest of the journal takes writers on a personal journey to examine what patterns in their lives prevent them from getting the things they want out of life or doing the things they want to do.

I strongly believe that our lives are richer and better if we can move toward an attitude of abundance. There really is more than enough to go around for everyone. There is plenty of wealth, jobs, houses, cars, love, peace, and health out there for all of us to have some. I may have breast cancer, but I can still walk, talk, see, breathe, think, go to the bathroom by myself, eat, scratch my itches, and enjoy the company of my lover and friends. By staying in a state of gratitude, I also stay in a place of empowerment where breast cancer is subservient to the way I choose to see it.

Throughout this book, I mention many paths that are possible, many perspectives, and many viewpoints. I can choose to focus on any one of them as a teacher. The academic part of me loves to look at the science of it all. I am easily mesmerized by the possibilities of stem cell transplants, smart chemotherapy drugs that kill only certain cells, the relationship between radiation therapy and cell death, plus myriad other complexities of cancers and their treatment. Within a few months of my last treatment, I met a woman who was diagnosed with stage four breast cancer and was still living two years later, teaching fulltime and enjoying her life, all as a result of a stem cell transplant. Without it, she would have been dead.

The spiritual part of me likes to explore what new connections I can make with God as a result of this disease. The philosophical and psychological parts of me like to explore different techniques for working with this disease in my body. The social activist part of me wants to help educate, activate, and debate the many potential causes of breast cancer. The political side of me wants to know why we still dump billions of dollars into killing people in war and demand that we spend an equal amount of money here on our soil, healing people. I believe the politico-spiritual paradox is that as long as we as a nation, or as humans on the same planet, stay invested in killing and committing heinous acts of violence, we will never have the collective resources to heal ourselves.

Healing requires a connected energy.   I wrote this book as an offering to that part of me that wants to educate and teach.   It is the book I wanted to read when I was going through this process. This book is not necessarily scientific in nature and it is not intended to be a self-help or guidance book, but it is a book about the journey. It is about the process of my ups and downs, and the ins and outs along the way. I wanted to know other people's stories when I was going through this process. I wanted to read how someone else did it without the pressure of having to attend a support group. Going to a support group seemed overwhelming at the time and just one more appointment to add to my already exhausted schedule.

Support groups are great tools for working with breast cancer and most cities have them. But sometimes just the solace of my own quiet space, not having to listen, respond, or take care of someone else, was a part of my journey. As a result, I cherished reading something with a little bit of emotion in it along with Susan Love's treatise on breast cancer.

But let me remind you that, just because I am choosing to look at my breast cancer through the lens of a teaching metaphor, I do not believe in any way that I caused my breast cancer. I think that's ludicrous! I know there is some literature on bookshelves that suggest that people who are sick somehow invite it into his/her life. I do not believe breast cancer is caused by what I ate or did not eat. I do not believe it is because

I grew up in a mill town where daily I washed the paper mill soot from the porch. I do not believe it is because I have a certain spiritual outlook rather than a different one. Cancer does not pick and choose deliberately. Neither I nor anyone I talk about in this book nor anyone I met along the way or anyone reading this book did something to invite cancer into their lives. We all are confronted with an assignment we never expected or encouraged. We must decide how we will respond to the demands physically, emotionally, and spiritually. In my life, once cancer and I became intimately connected, I had to decide how I wanted to handle this uninvited guest. Because literature helps me to make sense of my life, I sought for direction in my favorite books.

In *The Color Purple* Alice Walker provided me with ideals for my life. One lesson from that book that I try to practice daily is this: there are beautiful flowers in the world and I get to enjoy their brilliant colors. It is my recollection that the author creates a scene where Shug and Celie are walking through a meadow rich in the colors of spring. The two women have been each other's teachers, lovers and best friends throughout the toughest times. Shug says to Celie, "Don't you think God gets pissed when we don't even notice the flowers are purple?"

There is wonderful metaphoric power in this intimate discussion between the two women. Shug is indicating that the color purple should be noticed and marveled at just because it exists. Celie experiences an epiphany, a moment when she experiences that she, too, is to be noticed and marveled at just because she exists. In that moment, Celie connects with the color purple as her God. Nature begins to speak to her and through her. Later in the film, we find her speaking back to Albert, who has beaten and raped her, with words like, "A dust devil flew up on the porch between us, fill my mouth with dirt. The dirt say, Anything you do to me, already done to you. Then I feel Shug shake me. Celie, she say. And I come to myself. I'm pore, I'm black, I may be ugly and can't cook, a voice say to everything listening. But I'm here" (p. 207).

At that moment, Celie solidified her freedom.

Breast cancer was a similar epiphany moment for me. It amalgamated my freedom and propelled me to make the most out of my day and enjoy the richness of me. As Celie says, "I may be black, I may be poor, I may be ugly, but I am here."

Breast cancer awakened that "I Am Here" voice deep within me.

One lesson we all can learn from breast cancer, whether we have it or not, is that life as we know it is not forever. We have no guarantees of what comes next, so the art of living in the now is essential to our health and well-being. By looking at this disease through the lens of a teaching metaphor, I find myself asking, "What is it I believe about cancer, and how did I come to those beliefs? How does my own personal history impact my viewpoint about cancer?"

CHAPTER 14

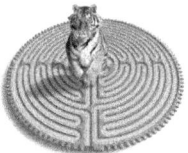

LESSONS FROM VIRGINIA

I said earlier in this book that I learned from my early childhood that cancer was a bad thing and it takes important people away from you, like it took Matt away from me. It wasn't until I was in my mid-twenties in my psychotherapy practice on Whidbey Island that I had the opportunity to learn and to heal from that early childhood belief that everyone who gets cancer dies of cancer. I had the wonderful life-changing experience as a therapist to work with a client by the name of Virginia. It was my therapeutic relationship with Virginia that taught me that not everyone who gets cancer dies of cancer. Sixty-five year old Virginia was short and round with bright red hair. She had a vivacious laugh that matched the constant twinkle in her eye. Virginia gave me her permission to use her name in this book. I met Virginia, an elementary teacher of thirty-six years, when I was working on Whidbey Island. For nineteen of those years she taught first grade. Virginia called me in August prior to her last year of teaching and inquired about my psychotherapy services. We scheduled a consultation and during the consultation, Virginia explained her goals. "I have taught all of my life. My identity is that of a first grade teacher, and I love those kids. But I want to retire and travel. I also want to find meaningful volunteer work to keep me active, involved, and alive on a daily basis."

I told her, "Virginia, if more people were like you, taking this transition seriously, doing the emotional work necessary to make an easy transition, the world would be a better place. I consider it an honor to be asked to accompany you on this journey."

She said, "During the night I have a lot of crazy dreams. Can you help me decipher their language?"

I explained, "I did quite a bit of dream work interpretation in my undergraduate program, and I work with my own dreams. There are several different angles that I can teach you to approach your dreams. One of the approaches that I like best is the story of the Senoi Indian tribe in South America, who are called the dream people. I understand that they live their daily life according to their nighttime dreams. We can start with that approach on your dream work and you can begin journaling your feelings about saying goodbye to a career you have loved."

We worked weekly that year on issues about family, time, loss, and making new goals. Virginia processed her many conflicting feelings and discovered the language of her nighttime dreams. I also taught her how to do visualization work or often called guided imagery. By the time her retirement date rolled around, she was less anxious and more secure about her new life. She was very excited about her new goals, incorporating various traveling plans throughout the next year while exploring different volunteer options. She continued her psychotherapy that summer after her retirement.

Summer was not quite over when I received a call. The male voice on the other end of the phone said, "I am calling to cancel Virginia's appointment next week. She is in the hospital having emergency surgery. The doctors think it is a ruptured appendix."

It was Virginia's husband, Vic. He went on to say, "She was at the base commissary when she began to have severe pain in her side. It did not let up, so she drove to the emergency room. They took her into emergency surgery. She asked me to call you as they were rolling her in."

I was concerned, but not terribly. Virginia was a really healthy lady and I knew she would be okay in the surgery.

Then two days later, Virginia called. "Robin, I want you to know I have colon cancer."

I got woozy with those words "colon cancer."

"No, Vic said you had a ruptured appendix." I said. All of us can say the most inane things when we are stressed.

"That is what we all were thinking. The pain was on my left side. It was sharp, and became increasingly worse. I broke out in a sweat from the pain by the time I arrived at the emergency room. But, when they opened me up, they discovered that a tumor had ruptured. It was attached to my colon, and it exploded inside of me," she explained.

I was swept with a cocktail of anger, sadness, and disbelief. Everything moved in slow motion. I managed, "Colon cancer, cancer cells all through your body. Virginia, I am sorry."

"I will be in the hospital for awhile and not able to drive for awhile. The doctors will be in to talk to me about what my options are in a few days," she said.

"Can I come to the base to see you?" I asked.

"I am too tired for visitors right now, maybe after a bit," she answered.

"Well, please keep me informed about what the doctors say. If you are not up to calling, please have Vic call." I floundered for words, any words.

"I will. I have to hang up now," she said.

"Goodbye, Virginia. Thanks for calling," I said.

I remember being as close to a rage as I had come in my life. I looked aimlessly around my surroundings. I just wanted something to throw as far and as hard as possible. Thankfully, I still had enough presence of mind not to throw anything. But the unfairness of it all enraged me. How can someone live their whole life, work hard, and even do their retirement right, and then get dealt this hand? This was some bad cosmic joke.

One day after visiting Virginia in the hospital, I pulled weeds in my flower garden. During that time, I had a long talk with God, and I knew I had to pull myself together and do what I needed to do. I needed to go through this tunnel with Virginia. I had to help her make this transition, too. During my undergraduate program, I had also studied the work of Elizabeth KublerRoss. Thus, I dug her books out of my personal library and refreshed my memory on the stages of death and dying. So, while Virginia recovered from her surgery, I re-read KublerRoss, bracing myself not to feel anything as I walked her to death's door. Elizabeth Kubler-Ross was the first in this country to address the inhumane ways we treat our terminally ill, especially how as a culture it seemed taboo to talk about the realities of death. Kubler-Ross created a template of the five stages of death. Those five stages are denial, anger, bargaining, depression, and finally acceptance. After reviewing the literature, I was now equipped with knowledge that allowed me to move far away from my feelings to my intellect. Intellectual armor is always very shiny, and my suit of armor fits me very well.

So, Virginia recovered from surgery, and she was told that there was no real treatment for her type of cancer. She was told that statistics suggested that her chance for survival were only twelve percent. However, the military base was conducting a study. Virginia fit the study protocol. The study was intriguing to her, but she wanted to talk to me first. Now with all of my intellectual armor, I am in favor of learning information that might help us make medical advances. But that is as long as the participants in those studies are no one I know. If the participants remain anonymous and faceless, I can review the study results protected, not having to imagine that anyone suffered or died as the result of the study.

About six weeks passed, Virginia drove to my office to begin working on this current issue - colon cancer. She came in, sat down, and said, "I have decided what I am going to do and I need you to help me."

"Sure, Virginia, anything you need," I said.

She pulled out a paperback book titled ***Getting Well Again.*** She said she had read it, and that she wanted to practice its visualization exercises in order to be an active participant in healing her body. It was in the next sentence that she explained the details of the above-mentioned study. She said, "I want to participate in medical science, but when I go to talk with them next Monday, I want them to understand that we are doing this visualization healing work; if they are concerned that it will taint the study, then I don't want to participate in the study."

She went on, "The study entails either receiving a new chemotherapy drug or a placebo. If I fall into the chemotherapy category, what if it makes me so sick that I can't do this visualization work?"

It was finally my turn. "Virginia, I know the study is important to you. It is just who you are. However, chemotherapy is designed to kill off your cells, healthy and unhealthy ones. Chemotherapy cannot discriminate between them. I do not know anyone who has had chemotherapy, but the reports that I have read about it paint a picture of nausea and discomfort. My question is, do you really want to subject yourself to that for experimental purposes?"

"Well, I know if I am drawn for that group it will be rough, but it just feels like the right thing to do. I will have to trust God to get chosen for the group He wants me in."

I was still pretty ticked off with God at this time and must have silently muttered, "If you can trust God to choose the right group, why can't he handle the big stuff, like not getting cancer at all?" Instead, I said, "Okay, then let's see what the study coordinator says about visualization as an active part of your treatment."

I was a young scrapper then, but not too young to know that no medical doctor was going to take visualization work seriously. Even at that time, I really did not take it all that seriously. I viewed is as a coping tool. And as far as I was concerned, Virginia's plan to do visualization was just a part of her doing stage three of the five stages of death and dying. Stage three, the bargaining stage, is where the patient hopes they can come up with some solution to postpone or delay death. For instance, when I was sixteen and in the hospital with pneumonia, I thought I was going to die. I bargained with God at that time. I prayed, "God, if you will just let me live I will get baptized as soon as I get out of the hospital." I lived and kept my promise much to my mother's distress. I was released from the hospital on Saturday and the next day I was baptized in full immersion in the water. Of course, at that time we thought wet hair caused the common cold that could turn into pneumonia. So for me, I nicely categorized Virginia's desire to do visualization work as part of the third stage of death and dying. At the end of our session time, Virginia said, "I would like for you to read this book."

It wasn't exactly a question. I told her, "Keep it and I will order me a copy."

She said, "I have a copy on order already. I've read this one through twice. I think the only thing I have to do now is come up with an image to use. In the book, they use the imagery of Pac-Man to go through the body and eat the mutant cells. I need to give it some more thought. That image doesn't work for me."

"Okay, Virginia. I will have the book finished by your next session. If you are seeing the doctors at the base on Monday, why don't you come in on Tuesday?"

I took the book home and read it. I must admit I really liked what it had to say. It was a perfect match for the visualization work I already taught. However, I still just had this underlying belief that everyone who gets cancer dies from cancer. I couldn't bring myself to trust in this method. I would use it with Virginia because even as a young psychotherapist, I was already an excellent and skilled therapist, and I knew enough to follow the client's lead, regardless of what I thought or believed. It is their work, their journey – not mine.

On the following Tuesday, I was equipped with some of the strategies from **Getting Well Again** and was struggling to place the third step of grief work, the bargaining stage, on default. Virginia came in all smiles and told me the doctor told her, "Certainly, you can practice whatever alternative technique you want. Especially since it is a mental technique, and you won't be putting anything in your body. It won't skew the results at all."

Virginia continued, "So, I signed up, and on Friday, I go to the base to draw for the study. Besides that, I have already come up with my image. I have started using the seven dwarfs and their song, Hi-ho, hi-ho', it's off to work we go. The book suggests twenty minutes, three times a day. I sit in my recliner and visualize Sleepy, Grumpy, and Sneezy getting their mops and mopping up all of my mutant cells, chasing them out through my urinary tract."

I was amazed at how quickly she had become entrenched in this process and amused by her first grade imagery. She really believed it and, thank God, she was not dependent on my belief at that time. In reality, Virginia did not really even need me. I was along for the ride because obviously the Universe had something to teach me. Virginia recovered fully from her colon cancer ordeal and went on to live a happy and healthy retirement.

In 1987, just before I moved to Arizona, I took a group from the Episcopal Church on Whidbey Island to Kenya. The purpose of the group was a socio-cultural mission to give them experiential education in actual outreach. The church on Whidbey gave a large percentage of its income to missions. Because of my background in missions work, I thought it would be an excellent way for me to say goodbye by taking a group to an actual hands-on experience and broaden their perception of the global church. There were eight total travelers: three adolescents, two of us middle-aged folks, and three seniors. And, you guessed it, Virginia was one of the seniors. At the time of this writing, Virginia was still living independently, traveling often, volunteering in her church library and ministering on the church's prayer chain. I saw her two years ago and she was in a retirement home, whirling around in her wheel chair, and telling me "Getting old is not for sissies."

For much longer than necessary, I continued to wait on her denial to end. But now, I can look back and say regardless of how her life ends, she had a wonderful and meaningful retirement.

There have been many stories in between my story and Virginia's story. One of the other seniors on the African trip died two years after the trip of stomach cancer. Another school teacher, who sought psycho-therapy with me because of my work with Virginia, died of lung cancer. I noticed that when this teacher was doing her visualization work there was a definite difference between her visualization and the one Virginia designed. The teacher who died always gravitated to comforting religious visualizations. She would see herself roller-skating with Jesus in a beautiful green park, and then when they were done roller skating, He would pour healing ointment all over her body, washing the cancer cells away. It was only after the fact – in hindsight – that my intellectual self could see the differences in the visualizations. Virginia's visualization was active, powerful and fun. The other visualization was passive and peaceful. But like I said, a good therapist follows the client's process and does not mess around with the client's imagery. I do believe clients know deep down inside of themselves, if they can only allow themselves to have access to that information. Virginia knew. I only thought I knew.

I did not know about either of their outcomes. I am just thankful that they did not need my belief system to make their visualizations powerful for them. Only now in reading this book might Virginia realize how scared I was at that time. What I do know **now** is that not everyone who gets cancer dies of cancer. So what about me?

I don't know yet.

CHAPTER 15

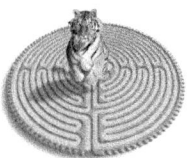

MORTALITY PUSHED OPEN THE DOOR

During my first few weeks of adjusting to my life with breast cancer, I lay awake at night trying to assimilate my new reality. In the whirlwind of this medical nightmare, I was no longer the person I used to be, and yet I could not identify what changed. I felt the same. I thought, *Yes, I have breast cancer; I am missing my right breast. I now have a scar starting under my right armpit running diagonally to the center of my chest. I know my body has changed, but how does that change me?*

This gnawing need to be able to identify what had changed just wouldn't let up.

I tried to remember that breast cancer was not the worst thing in the world. Many people suffer worse than this every day in our country, not to mention those in third world countries.

I hate it when my clients use that last line. When clients say to me, "Even though I was physically and sexually abused, my abuse was not as bad as other kids."

I tell them, "That might be true, but you are the one in my office right now and it is your story that is important to me."

But between the hours of two to four early in the morning, I was perturbed, as I tried to figure out what was different. I could not articulate what had changed. What was this difference?

Then it came to me. In the book *Journey to Ixtlan*, Don Juan taught Carlos Castaneda a lesson -- a lesson that bothered me the first time I read it. Even before reading the book, I had read an excerpt from *Journey to Ixtlan* in the book *Soul Making* by Allan Jones. Don Juan, a Yaqui Indian Shaman, had a very eager student, Carlos Castaneda. One day, Don Juan and Castaneda went hunting for rabbits. Don Juan was explaining to Castaneda that he would have to trap, kill, skin, cook, and eat the rabbit. That did not seem like a big deal to Castaneda because he liked to hunt. He had hunted most of his life. But on this day, something different happened. The rabbit was lured into the cage, causing the rabbit great panic. Castaneda approached the cage; the rabbit stared directly into Castaneda's eyes, penetrating his soul.

"Don Juan then gave the command, 'Now kill it.' Castaneda put his hands into the trap and grabbed the rabbit by the ears. Castaneda's terror suddenly seized him. He dropped the rabbit back into the cage and refused to kill it. Don Juan turned his ferocious eyes on Castaneda, and with all the force of his authority repeated his command, 'Kill it'" (pp. 75-79).

It was the rabbit's time to die. This was the moment. Still Castaneda refused. This time Don Juan yelled at him. The rabbit has to die.

Castaneda goes on: "A series of confusing thoughts and feelings overtook me, as if the feelings had been out there waiting for me. I felt with agonizing clarity the rabbit's tragedy, to have fallen into my trap. In a matter of seconds my mind swept across the crucial moments of my life, the many times I had been the rabbit myself. I looked at it and it looked at me. The rabbit had backed up against the side of the cage. We exchanged a somber glance, and that glance, which I fancied to be one of silent despair, cemented a complete identification on my part. 'The hell with it,' I said loudly. 'I won't kill anything. The rabbit goes free.' Castaneda panicked. He tried to grab the rabbit by the ears to set the creature free. By this time the rabbit was so terrified that it moved out of reach. Castaneda became desperate, and in frustration tried to break the trap. He kicked the trap as hard as he could. At all costs that rabbit was to run free again. The trap would not break. So with a supreme effort he brought his right foot down on the corner of the trap with tremendous force. The wood broke, and he grabbed the rabbit with relief. But it remained motionless in his hand. It was dead. Don Juan stared at Castaneda. The brujo put his hand on his pupil's head and whispered in his ear. He had not completed his task. The rabbit had still to be skinned, roasted, and eaten. Castaneda felt sick to his stomach" (pp. 75-76).

I had felt that same sick feeling several times during this journey. I felt sick when I looked at my scar. I felt sick when I thought too far ahead to what might happen to me. I was finally able to put my finger on what makes me different now. Like Castaneda, death had become my constant advisor. That powerful story wrapped up the following lessons for me, explained by Jones in **Soul Making**. *"The rabbit's tragedy was his own, and yet the rabbit's death was a gift not to be wasted just as his death would be a gift to someone else. Acceptance of this gift depended on Castaneda's ability to set aside his own sense of importance. The receiving of such gifts requires some kind of dying to self. As we have seen, the feeling of dread disappears when such gifts are accepted… I am convinced, however, that something positive begins to happen within me when I do look death, my death, straight in the eye. Death puts my whole being into question without being able to answer the question. I have to surrender to the uncertainty of death, and this surrender can be simply an act of despair in the ultimate futility of being."* (p.77).

On page 74 of **Soul Making** we find the truth that Don Juan was teaching Castaneda: "Death, then, is our constant companion. It is the only advisor we have. Whenever you feel, as you always do, that everything is going wrong and you are about to be annihilated, turn to your death and ask if it is so. Your death will tell you that you're wrong; that nothing really matters outside of its touch. Your death will tell you, 'I haven't touched you yet.' As we live into the truth of this, our dread is transformed into our delight. Sister Death, as St. Francis calls her, challenges us to live life as fully and as creatively as we can."

I realized in those wee hours of early morning that death had indeed become my constant companion. I now had the experience to go with my philosophical belief. I had to learn to balance the scales between death, my advisor, and the inner warrior who was bound and determined to beat the statistics.

CHAPTER 16

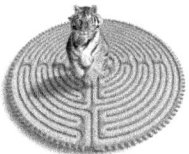

THE VIRGIN BRINGS IN THE TIGERS

With Virginia's success and Castaneda's story burning fire in my soul, I knew visualization was the tool I needed to help my body heal. I also knew it was imperative that I find a way to work from a place of detachment versus a place of fear. What images would help me do that?
This work is very spiritual to me. I consider myself a spiritual person and use lots of symbols and rituals in my daily spiritual practice. I have a home altar and one in my therapy office. I keep significant Christian symbols, special art, rosaries, candles, and many Native American tools to assist me in my daily walk. Regardless, of all of the symbolism I utilize, my Christian connection is my strongest. The story and power of Christ are very real for me; thus I was not surprised when I had this very powerful thought zap across my brain, "I really need to go to the top here," and it made sense to me that the Mother of God was as far up in the chain of authority as one can go.

The Mother of God, a woman and a historical figure whose story has been carried down from generation to generation, just like the story of Christ, seemed to be the most powerful person I could appeal to during this time of need. However, I never really thought much about the Mother of God until breast cancer knocked at my door. Perhaps choosing the symbol of the Mother of God was one way to reconnect with my own mother, who was deceased and who I missed very much. Catholics and Episcopalians use the rosary, a group of connected beads, to pray to the Mother of God. I often carry my rosary with me when I am seeking guidance about something, or praying for something or someone in particular. The beginning of the rosary prayer is "Hail Mary, full of grace. Blessed art thou among women. Blessed is the fruit of your womb, Jesus. Hail Mary, Mother of God, pray for me now and at the hour of my death." The death word was uncomfortable to me and still is. Instead, I pray, "Hail Mary, Mother of God, pray for me now and always."

I also sought another image to work directly in the actual visualization work. I prayed, "Mother of God, bring me an image I can truly believe in; an image that will empower me and help me fight my fear as I use that image to help me heal."

I understood deep down inside that I needed to confront this lesson, look it square in the eye, and abolish my fear. It is my professional opinion that fear drives anxiety, and anxiety and fear undermine the power of visualization work.

One night in twilight sleep I looked over at my bedroom door. I saw a tiger sitting there in a holy opulence. It was yellow with black stripes. I knew instantly that my ally had arrived to help me heal. I began my meditation/visualization process. It doesn't really matter what you call it; what is important is how it is used.

In a previous chapter I mentioned that one of my innate scripts or beliefs is that people who get cancer die of cancer. That belief was intertwined deep within my psyche. That was what I believed in my core self. I wasn't going to stop believing that by just chanting or reciting that all people who get cancer do not die of cancer. Belief systems don't work that way. If I started saying to myself, "Not all people who get cancer die of cancer," then I would be lying to myself.

It is important how we phrase language. Our brain does not compute double negatives well. A sentence like "Not all people who get cancer die of cancer" is computed as, "All people who get cancer die of cancer." The brain does not compute the "not" at the beginning. Thus, sentence structure needs to be in active voice, such as, "The tigers are eating my mutant cells, making my body whole." The psyche has an internal system that works very hard to get our lives to be congruent.

Congruency means that our outside life matches our inside life, and vice versa. When we lie to ourselves with what some behavioral therapists call positive affirmation, our psyche screams out "liar!" Our psyche counteracts the affirmation and a very unnecessary internal battle takes place. As far as I know, no one has ever lost weight by standing in front of the mirror and saying five, ten, or twenty times a day, "I am thin."

Affirmations were a good idea in the Seventies and Eighties, but they were not very effective. Many psychotherapy clients "failed therapy" because, regardless of how many times they tried using those affirmations, nothing happened. Some clients left therapy feeling worse instead of better. Today, we understand more about how the brain works and synthesizes information. Today guided imagery, affirmations, and visualization are structurally worded so that the brain can process and use their power for the benefit of the client.

Visualization is a process that helps us access all of our body and each of our sensory contact points. Four primary ways that each of us learn about ourselves and the environments we live in are through our visual, auditory, kinesthetic and proprioceptive channels. The big difference between proprioceptive information and kinesthetic information is the difference between body movement (kinetic) and body awareness (proprioceptive). The proprioceptive channel deals with our breathing, eyelid movement, stomach, internal sensations, and feelings of body pressure; the kinesthetic channel deals with our body movement, such as hand, leg movement, touch, texture, and how our body moves in response to what is going on in the environment. When visualizations are designed appropriately, they touch each of those areas, aligning everything in your body, making everything congruent.

In other words, I might not believe that I can heal myself from cancer, but I did believe that my ally, the tiger, had the power to eat my mutant cells. The tiger goes through my body, gobbles up the mutant cells, and then escapes with those cells through my toes. I used my toes as the exit route because I didn't want any residual cancer cells in my urinary tract.

The visual work I did and still do looks like this. I see the molecular *in vitro* baby cells of tigers enter my Groshong, the surgically implanted catheter for my chemotherapy, and come through the tube into my body. As soon as the tigers hit my blood stream, they awaken and begin maturing. Thousands of baby tigers patrol every molecular area in my body looking for ugly, mean little mutant cells. The tigers gobble up the mutant cells as soon as they see them. The more mutant cells the baby tigers eat, the larger the tiger becomes. When the tigers complete their search, they come roaring out of my toes. For days after finishing chemotherapy, and even now, I visualize the same thing again activating my tigers to keep working on my behalf.

I use all of my senses to create a reality. It is easy for me to smell the tigers because they have a distinctively strong and not very pleasant odor. Their odor became an intricate part of my reality because the chemotherapy exuded a very unpleasant odor from my pores. Once I am aware of the smell of the tigers, I hear them breathe deeply, and then snarl, making growling noises as they go after the mutant cells. When they come running out of my toes, they go to a faraway place to urinate the mutant cells out of their body, lick themselves clean, and take a nap – all normal cat behavior. When I call for them the next morning, they return to me transformed as infant tiger cells awaiting their mission.

The Groshong was surgically implanted into my subclavian vein just below the collar bone. The tip of the Groshong lies in the large vein that returns blood to the heart. Whether I was in a chemotherapy session or not, I continued to see these *in vitro tiger* cells enter through the catheter. When the Groshong was removed, it left a scar. Thus, it was natural to see the tigers entering through the scar on my remaining breast, into my heart, and into the blood system to begin their maturation process. Eleven years later, I still invite my tiger allies to return and keep my body free of mutant cells. Today, I invite the tigers by kissing my tiger necklace as I place it around my neck, then I gently close my eyes and invite the tigers to come and do their work.

It is my understanding that all of us have mutant cells in our bodies to some degree. This is not particularly harmful unless those cells find each other. If they do find each other, they attach themselves to each other, creating a tumor. The tumor then grows by tapping into our nutrient-filled blood system. Medically, it is a bit more complicated, but I am attempting to provide a visual that is easy to grasp. Once an image makes sense, it is easy to construct a visualization exercise that is helpful. I do believe that by finding an ally to go into to your body, whether it is tigers, the seven dwarfs, or any of a myriad of other images or symbols, you are working with your body, helping it to heal. I've included a few good books in the reference section that might be useful to you in this process.

CHAPTER 17

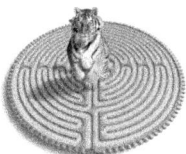

TIGER HISTORY AND CHOOSING MY PERSONAL SYMBOLS

When the tiger appeared to me that night in my bedroom doorway, I was neither surprised nor confused by the symbol. The tiger has been a very meaningful symbol to me all of my life. I have a baby picture of me when I am less than two months old; one of the identifiable toys lying in the crib with me is a stuffed tiger sitting near my head. The only Halloween costume I remember is a tiger costume which, I think, was more likely a pair of pajamas with feet. It had a very long tail and I wore it trick-or-treating when I was very young.

I recall that my favorite book was **Little Black Sambo**. I am aware this book has been controversial over the years, but obviously I was engrossed by the tigers in the book and at the age of three or four, I was unaware of the politics of race. Besides, Matt my caregiver was black. The book has now been republished in a politically correct manner and renamed *The Story of Little Babji*. But when I was little my version of the book was about an East Indian child, whose mother made him bright and beautiful clothes. When he went for a walk in the jungle, the tigers threatened to eat him if he didn't give them a piece of his beautiful clothes. After about five times of continual tiger harassment, poor Little Black Sambo was naked. As he tried to find his way home, he heard a loud, discontented growling noise. At first, he was very afraid because he thought the tigers had not kept their word and were going to eat him anyway. But as he peered around the bush he was hiding behind, he saw the strangest thing. In their greed to get all of Little Black Samba's clothing, they had hold of each others' tails and they would not let go. They were chasing each other, circling a tree. The tigers became so hot and so tired, they turned into a pool of melted butter, and Little Black Sambo made it home safely. When his father arrived home that evening, he brought home a container full of fresh butter. Little Black Sambo's mother fixed pancakes for dinner and the three of them enjoyed the pancakes with the butter. Little Black Sambo was mesmerized as he ate his pancakes because he had never seen butter with black stripes.

I don't remember much more about the tiger until my adult life. While living on Whidbey Island, I wrote a poignant poem about a tiger mother. I subsequently did some research on tigers and discovered they are very maternal, keeping watch and protecting their young for two years after birth.

I began my doctorate work a few years after I arrived in Phoenix. During that time, I attended a workshop facilitated by a good friend and colleague of mine, Dr. Judy O'Donoghue. The workshop was an experiential Stanislav Grof holotropic breath-work workshop. As a participant, I lay on a mat on the floor and was instructed to breathe very fast and deep to the very loud and intense music that was playing in the background. As I followed the instructions, I began to hear my own deep breathing, and I began to feel my body "joggle up and down." My imagination was activated and I imagined that I was an unborn baby tiger in my mother's womb. I was sloshing gently back and forth in embryonic fluid. I was aware that my tiger mother was running up a mountain in unfamiliar territory. At the time, I just assumed it was a mountain in India. When the tiger arrived at the top of the mountain, she found a tree and dug around it, making room for my birth. The next thing I knew, I was pushed through this tunnel, and soon after felt my mother's tongue licking me. Her tongue tickled. I felt an overwhelming sense of being loved. I knew I had experienced my birth. I was a tiger. The tickling from her tongue licking me brought me back to my normal state of reality, and I awakened on the mat on the floor. Two hours had elapsed when I felt like it had only been a few minutes. I do not believe this is a past life experience, nor was it intended to be. I believe that my soul identifies with the tiger. Carl Jung spoke about this in his impressive work on symbols and archetypes.

It wasn't until late 1998, when I was ready to publish a journal for clients, *Writing Your Way to Healing and Wholeness*, that I noticed the tiger again. I was looking for a background for the journal pages – a watermark as it's referred to in the printing industry. I was limited to the art in my computer, which is considered archaic these days. It was a toss-up between a picture of hot air balloons or the tiger. I chose the tiger, for no specific reason at that time, except that I liked it. It was a few months into my chemotherapy that I picked up that journal and realized there was the tiger staring back at me.

You may want to search for your symbols and images as a result of reading this chapter. In order to do that, allow yourself to take an inventory of the stories in your life; see if you have a recurrent image running through them. Let your history advise your present and complement your future.

For instance, my tiger is an image that has been consistently present in my history. I can now see from the crib to my book *Writing Your Way to Wholeness*, the tiger has been there. Now I use its symbolism to help me negotiate my present which will help me in my future.

CHAPTER 18

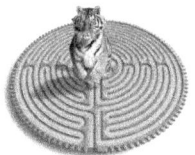

THE LONG RIDE

By the time of my second oncology visit with Dr. Langford, my anxiety shriveled and I noticed that he really did not talk like Donald Duck. My second appointment with him was September 13, 1999, my first day of chemotherapy. On the 7th of September, I finished all of my testing, the CT scan, bone scan, and lung x-ray. On the 9th of September, I had another outpatient surgery to "install" a Groshong, a central line going into my left breast and straight to my heart in order that the chemotherapy could be delivered to my body in the exact location. The Groshong would keep my veins from being burned or collapsing from the constant poking and multiple insertions of needles for blood work and chemotherapy. It became amusing to watch nurses try to get my blood draws from my Groshong. It was not nearly as easy as they had hoped. My veins were and are much more co-operative, but I am sure my veins are thankful they did not have to suffer the abuse.

On that day, September 13, Dr. Langford and I spoke for a few minutes. I don't recall any of what he said, but I became aware that the protocol is to always meet with him prior to the chemotherapy treatment. During all future pre-chemotherapy appointments, he asked a lot of questions: How are you feeling? Are you having any side effects? How is the Zophran (anti-nausea drug) working for you? Are you experiencing nausea or weight loss?

Then his nurse took me into the treatment room. Prior to the first treatment, I peeked into the treatment room. It was the typical muted colors of beige and green, the walls lined with recliner chairs. I don't believe there was any art on the walls. If there was, it sure was not interesting art. I usually chose a recliner facing the windows. That helped some. Pam always went with me. I would take a few quiet moments to load my tigers on board, and then she and I talked to each other. Most patients didn't talk to each other, and we all did our best not to look at each other. There were eight to ten recliners, maybe even as many as twelve. On this first day all of them were full, except the one waiting for me. I sat in it.

The nurse took my blood pressure, which back then was always normal regardless of my internal stress. She went over some instructions with me and again informed me that I would be given two chemotherapy drugs during these first four treatments and a different chemotherapy drug for the last four treatments. The first two chemotherapy drugs were Adriamycin and Cytoxan. I remember them based on how I learned to pronounce them. I was administered Adriamycin first. It was red, Kool-Aid red. It was dispensed by the nurse with a large syringe. The nurse was careful not to let any of it drip on her or me. If Adriamycin touches the bare skin, it will burn. There is nothing like trying to relax and invite tigers to be born in the chemotherapy drug when your awareness rises to meet reality, whispering, "Now, Robin, they are going to put powerful poisons in your body." And I was supposed to believe this was a good thing!

Adriamycin is the drug responsible for the hair loss. And by the way, hair loss means all of the hairs all over your body, not just the hair on your head. Not only do you lose your hair with Adriamycin, the other side effects can be nausea, vomiting, and mouth ulcers. It suppresses the elements of the bone marrow including the white cells and platelets. It accumulates in the body, thus only small doses are given. If too much is administered, it can damage the heart. Cytoxan is similar.

I didn't ask but my guess is that I received both because Cytoxan is not as heavy a hitter as Adriamycin, and because the body can only tolerate so much of the Adriamycin. I was told to drink lots of water and I was given anti-nausea medication through the Groshong and a prescription for Zophran to take the next three to four days. The nurse also told me that my urine would be red for a couple of days, but the more water I drank the quicker I would be able to flush the poison from my system.

After the nurse finished pumping the Adriamycin into my Groshong, she hooked me up to the IV drip which contained the Cytoxan. I believe each of the above chemotherapy treatments took from two to two and a half hours. It was a very surreal experience to sit in a recliner designed for relaxing and watching TV, and willingly submit my body to poisons while watching everyone else do exactly the same thing. I wanted to scream, "Let me out of this nightmare. My God, are we all nuts?"

But I never let out that scream or any other reaction. I was a good soldier.

Every third week I would return and go through this process all over again. I always wondered who would be in the chemotherapy room. I wondered if those people who had chemo three weeks ago were still alive. I wondered too, *will I live to see the end of treatment? What types of cancers did other people have?* One guy had lung cancer. That was clear by the oxygen tank that came with him. He was around my age. Pam saw his obituary in the paper not too long after I completed my treatment.

Pam and I met and actually talked with a younger woman whose breast cancer had returned and was in her bones. She seemed optimistic. I don't know if she is still alive or not. Reading obituaries is not necessarily what I recommend, but if you do read the obituaries you will notice fatalities of people thirty and forty years old with no explanation of death. Sometimes you will get a hint of how they died when the family wants the donations to go to one of the cancer societies. I think we may have talked to one other guy during the whole six months of chemotherapy. Everyone in the room was dealing with their own fear, shame, and discomfort in the best way they knew how and hearing how things are going with others seemed to be too risky.   It is sometimes easier not to know.

After the first treatment, we stopped by Walgreen's to have my anti-nausea drug unsuccessfully filled. Then we came home. My friend Karen's mother, Helen, had fixed split pea soup for us and they dropped it by. I noticed I felt hyper and a bit odd. I had an awful taste in my mouth that brushing my teeth didn't help. Then I had to pee. Bright red urine filled the toilet. It was eerie and scary. I ate a bit of soup and drank some juice before I went to bed. The night was uneventful. The next day I went to work as usual. I didn't miss a day of work during those first four chemotherapy treatments.

By the third week after my first treatment, it was time to shave my head. My hair dresser stayed late on a Saturday to perform the shave in privacy.   I am very fortunate because my head is perfectly round, and thus bald was very becoming to me. It took others awhile to adjust to my sporty new bald look. I wasn't quite prepared when my pubic hair also left its home. Losing that hair was much more difficult for me than shaving my head. Somehow it made me feel less like a woman and again like a vulnerable little girl who couldn't grow up and be a woman. That accentuated any negative feelings I had about myself and my woman-hood.

I don't remember too much about the weeks in between treatment. There was never enough time after a treatment to emotionally prepare for the next one. The ten days post treatment is known as nadir. Nadir is the time when your blood count is at its lowest before it starts coming back. If it is too low during that time, they will give you a shot of Neupogen in order to boost the immune system and jump start cell growth. So halfway between treatments I would have to go back to the doctor's office and get my blood drawn. It wasn't until Taxol that I had to have injections of Neupogen I noticed I was more tired than usual, but never so exhausted that I couldn't work.   During treatment I saw no new clients, but continued to see my existing client load. Thus my schedule thinned out over the months of treatment and I was able to lie down on the office floor and sleep during breaks or cancellations.

CHAPTER 19

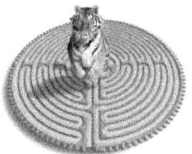

A VISIT FROM FAMILY

I made it through the first four treatments, feeling a bit like chemo-therapy was a piece of cake. Not once did I throw up, perhaps due to the drug Zophran. I continued to work and by Thanksgiving I was through with the Adriamycin/Cytoxan regimen. Pam and I went to the cabin as we had in the past over Thanksgiving. I was bald. We did what we normally do at the cabin which was eat, sleep, read, watch TV and walk – mostly in that order, too.

The following weekend, my cousin Linda Carol was coming to visit. Only a few of my family members have ever visited me in Arizona. I suspected that Linda Carol was coming because she thought I was go-ing to die. I am not sure and never braved the question, but I do know cancer has a way of making life more meaningful and nudging people to do things that they have put off. When Linda Carol came I took her, my bald head, and all to do the touristy things in Arizona.

First we went to Sedona to spend the night. We arrived on a cold Fri-day afternoon, taking our time to stop and take pictures of the red rock formations along the way. Shortly after arriving, we booked a Pink Jeep Tour for that afternoon. I visit Sedona often but had never bothered to take n a Pink Jeep Tour. I always suspected they were a sham. But because it was Christmas and quite chilly, the Pink Jeep Tour seemed like a reasonable way to see the red rock up close and personal. I must confess, both Linda Carol and I were very impressed. The tour was very informative while the four-wheeling was exquisite. The highlight of the four-wheeling was near the end of the tour when the jeep crept down a narrow embankment of stone-like steps. We were literally at a 90-degree angle. Linda Carol and I held on, held our breath, and giggled like school girls, keeping our eyes shut. We had a great time and have some incredible photos to prove it.

Because it was the first weekend in December, Sedona's marvelous Christmas light display was open. But before the two of us took off to get into the Christmas spirit we topped off our jeep ride with an elegant dinner at the Cowboy Club. With a name like the Cowboy Club, we weren't quite sure it would live up to its advertising, but thought we would give it a try. It was awesome. I had fresh halibut which they say they fly in fresh daily. It was sweet and moist, melting in my mouth. It didn't have any fishy taste, so they must have flown it in fresh. I am trying hard to eat more fish as the omega 3s are supposed to be good for me, but fish is not something I yearn for. Linda Carol ordered the duck. I just have never been able to quite get up the courage to try duck. I had a bite of hers and it was very tender, and not gamey. However, I still pass on it at restaurants. For the fun of the touristy thing we ordered the fried cactus appetizers. They came with a jalapeno dip. Then we finished off the evening with a spectacular chocolate and raspberry desert with chocolate ice cream. Isn't it amazing that I can be sitting here at my computer years later and recall to the "t" what we ordered that night for dinner?

After dinner we bundled up in jackets, gloves, and hats and rode the trolley to the L'Auberge Christmas display. Christmas lights bring out the child in me. I find them magical, mystical and a delight in their ability to make me smile. These light displays were above and beyond what I expected. Linda Carol and I were transfixed by some of scenes, especially the animated scenes where the snowman moved or the Disney characters danced. "Gee, Linda Carol, I am so glad you came to visit. I see this light display advertised every year, but have never driven up here to see it," I said.

"Well, Robin, I just don't think I will be able to explain to the folks back home how exhilarating these lights are, or the red rock for that matter. I just don't think the camera is going to catch the magnitude of it all," she said.

"Yes, this display is particularly awesome," I continued as we walked by a Santa Claus and his elves.

We spent a couple of hours walking around and looking at the light displays. I couldn't help but think about my mother when Linda Carol was here. She and my mom were very close. The only time my mother ever came to visit me, Linda Carol and my sister-in-law Jeannie came with her when I lived in Washington. They stayed for ten days and we went everywhere, including a day trip to Canada. I have fond memories of taking my mother around the different sites in Washington State. As the lights twinkled and Christmas music filled the background, I found myself wondering how much my mother would have enjoyed Arizona.

See, I was raised in a little mill town in the southwest mountains of Virginia, a range called the Alleghanies. I grew up with cousins, playing in the creek, hanging out at the playground, catching balls, and going one-on-one at the lonely basketball hoop. Life stood still when I was a child, making everything around me safe, secure, and innocent. There were no gangs, no drive-by shootings, and not very many keg parties.

My mother had flown only once prior to her trip to Washington. I had accompanied her on the previous trip to Italy, where we traveled to be with Valerie, the sole surviving grandchild, after a lethal car accident that took the lives of my oldest brother, his wife and the younger niece, Martine. Coming to visit me in Washington State was her first leisure trip and the very first flight for Linda Carol and Jeannie, too. My mother died shortly after I moved to Arizona. With the magic of Christmas in the air and the worry of death by cancer in my head, I sure was missing my mamma. Having Linda Carol here brought up all of those nostalgic feelings as well as amplified the reality that I didn't have a mom that I could talk to about my scary feelings. I wondered what comforting words my mother would have to say to me about my cancer, as well as how she might have worried herself sick. My mother did have an excessive worry gene that kept her all tied up in knots most of her life. Thankfully, I didn't get too much of that gene. I knew my mother would want me to be okay. I knew she would encourage me, reminding me like she did when I was a child, "You can do anything you set your mind to."

It is that type of tenacity that helps me fight this thing and get through it and other battles in my life. Maybe it is those words that have encouraged me to be where I am in my life today.

The silence between Linda Carol and me was profound. The nostalgia of Christmas memories long past, filled up the space between us where no words were needed to reunite the family bond and stories we shared. The cold air, the windy jeep ride, the excitement of being together again worked its magic, tuckering us out. Soon we called it a day.

The next day we were up early and out the door to a place called Jerome. Jerome is a little old copper town that is one of the several "artistic pockets" of Arizona. The people who live there are interesting folk, the landscape is mountainous and extraordinarily green, and the art is actually quite praiseworthy. Linda Carol was able to purchase a painting of Sedona she liked and have it shipped to her home.

Then we had lunch at a local place that was humming with activity, and over lunch she asked a few questions, like, "What has chemotherapy been like for you?"

I shared with her, "Chemotherapy has been very different than what I expected. The Zophran keeps me from throwing up and I still have quite a bit of energy. The hardest part for me right now is going into that room of recliners where other people are receiving their treatment. It is emotionally draining to have to be confronted with the hard cold facts that some of them won't be alive next year."

"Are you feeling good about your treatment?" she asked.

I knew that was a question about whether I thought I would be alive a year from now. It was in the answer that I took the time to talk with her about the "tigers" and the visual work that I do on a daily basis. I told her it was in that work that I was able to remain positive. I summarized the story about the visualization by saying, "I know I don't have all of the control in the world over the outcome of this, but I do want to have control over the parts that I can. I really do believe that by working with myself in this way I am increasing my odds. It is important for me to be able to look back at this and say, 'Hey I did my share.'"

"Your mother would be proud of how well you are handling this," she said.

"Your visit really makes me miss her more than I have in a long time," I responded.

We both teared up a bit and then the inevitable happened. "Would you like anything else?" the waitress interrupted.

"No, we're ready for the check," I said.

And then we distracted ourselves by returning to less emotional discussions. I drove her the long way down the mountain from Jerome. We picked up Pam and the three of us drove off to meet friends for the Phoenix Christmas Light Parade. We perched in the back of their pickup truck, drank hot chocolate, and tried to stay warm while, once again, the mood of Christmas made me wonder, *Will I be here, next year?*

Linda Carol flew back to the South, and I prepared for a new chemo drug called "Taxol."

CHAPTER 20

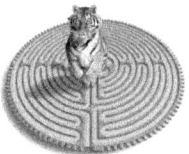

THE TAXOL EXPERIENCE

Monday came soon enough. My treatment was at 11:00 a.m.

I was in and out of my Cytoxan and Adriamycin treatments within three hours, but Taxol was a five-hour treatment. Pam joined me at Dr. Langford's office. After my brief checkup, I was once again advised of the multitude of dangers from Taxol with all of its potential side effects. I was quickly entering that space of oxygen deprivation; everything in the room was becoming very surreal. I was scared to death.

Dr. Langford informed me again, "Your fingers and toes may become numb or tingly from nerve damage caused by the Taxol."

Next we went to the chemotherapy room. The nurse sat down with a handful of consent forms and said, "Some people have an allergic reaction to the drug, which can be lethal. You will know immediately if you are having a reaction. You won't be able to breathe. We have the oxygen tank right here if that happens. We will stop the drug immediately. You will be provided with oxygen while the paramedics are in-route. They will then take you to the hospital."

So much for the Taxol taking my breath away, by the time she was finished with her informed consent statement my lungs were stuck to the inside of my chest wall, hiding out of abject fear. I was thinking, *Just let me have a little of that oxygen now!*

I signed the consent forms which I am sure I could battle in court as "not in my right mind." Being in stark naked terror and bottomless fear does have a way of taking control of my mental capacities and rendering me incompetent, doesn't it?

The drip was started and within five minutes, I was able to relax into the tiger visualization realizing that the window of fear had passed. I had no allergic reaction to the drug. But still today, as predicted, the very tips of my fingers are numb, which isn't a problem. However, my toes are numb and tingly on both feet all the way to the pads beneath the toes. This becomes uncomfortable at times.

Taxol is an interesting chemotherapy drug. Taxol (Paclitaxol) is a diterpenoid taxane derivative found in the bark and needles of the western yew, *Taxus Brevifolia*, indigenous to the old growth forests of the Pacific Northwest. The yew is a slow growing bush from the Evergreen family. It contains a mixture of alkaloids known as taxane, as well as diterpenes (including Taxol in some varieties), lignans, tannin and resin. In history, the yew tree was sacred to the Druids, who are believed to have considered it an emblem of immortality.

So what does Taxol actually do? Taxol inhibits cell division. Thus, the cells die off and are rendered powerless to create new ones. On this first treatment that information didn't mean a whole lot to me. My former chemotherapies had been uneventful. I had become accustomed to thinking that I would breeze through these Taxol treatments, too. The first day I seemed fine after the treatment.

That evening I still seemed fine, so I began to assume that all was going well with the Taxol. But in the middle of the night, I began to hurt. First, my back hurt, then my legs, especially my upper thighs began to rivet with pain. I took Ibuprofen. I called Langford's office the next day reporting the unbearable pain. He called in a prescription of Percocet. The Percocet went in and within thirty minutes the Percocet came out. I vomited for the first time since I had begun treatment. My body handled the poisons with the help of the anti-nausea drugs, but no way was my body going to tolerate the Percocet. My stomach rebelled. Morphine was prescribed for the next treatment. Nothing helped. The pain lasted about three days. I believed I was able to actually feel the cell inhibition. The pain mimicked what I imagined was happening in my body. I figured my cells were going about their business doing what cells do, which was to divide and multiply. Yet, like a burglar in the middle of the night, the Taxol attacked them, threw a hood over them, and bound and gagged them. They could not divide. The harder they tried to free themselves, the tighter the Taxol grip became, snuffing the very life right out of them. After about three days they give up the battle and my body began to relax and to recover from the torture. However, it was a hell of a fight those cells put up for three solid days.

With my second Taxol treatment, I missed my very first day of work as a result of chemotherapy. I was of no use to any of my clients. Nothing helped my pain and I was miserable. I couldn't focus, think, or sit comfortably. I stayed home and flipped the television from one channel to the next waiting for this three-day sentence to expire.

By my third treatment I found a natural remedy that seemed to help some, but not to the degree I'd hoped it would. Also, by my third treatment, my white cell count dropped so low that I was given injections of Neupogen. Neupogen is an Amgen product given by injection (don't cringe – remember my Groshong port – I felt nothing) to boost my white cell count. Procrit, which most of you have seen advertised ("I am too tired to do my daughter's wedding dress") builds red blood cells while Neupogen builds white blood cells. I needed all of the white cells I could get to help me beat this cancer. Remember, you were taught in elementary school that red cells make a body healthy and full of energy and white cells fight off infection. You see, the whole concept of chemotherapy is quite paradoxical. I was given poisons to kill cells. But when my cell count went down too far, I was given other drugs to raise my cell count to within normal ranges again. It sure doesn't make a lot of sense, but I supposed trying to find the perfect balance between life and death is in and of itself a paradox.

With the injections for my white blood cells and some natural pain relief, I finished up the eighth round of chemotherapy. I remember that on the tenth day (nadir) after my last treatment, when I walked back to my car after finishing with chemotherapy for what I hoped was forever, I shed my first set of tears since the day I was told, "I am surprised, but the cancer has invaded eight of twelve of your lymph nodes."

Chemotherapy was over and I was crying in the middle of the parking lot by my car. My insides heaved with turbulent emotions, emotions that I was not sure that I ever took the opportunity to fully understand. I supposed part of the turbulence was relief that I had lived through the process.

The other part of the overwhelming emotions was that emotional let-down that comes when "it" (whatever "it" might be) is finally over. The other feelings, more complex and rooted in fear, echoed questions like, *Did it work? Will I be okay now? What am I supposed to do next to keep the cancer at bay? "It is up to me and the tigers now. What if we fail?*

Of course I wasn't really finished. I still had thirty-three sessions of radiation therapy to complete, which I was still not fully convinced was the best option for me.

CHAPTER 21

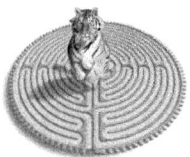

RADIATION TREATMENT

Radiation therapy is the use of high-energy ionizing rays to treat cancer. Radiation is used to treat cancer because the beams interfere with the ability of cells, both cancerous and healthy, to grow and multiply. Radiation in mega doses causes extreme mutations, like those seen after the bombing of Hiroshima during World War II. Radiologists, x-ray technicians, and dental patients wear a protective shield when giving or receiving radiation. It is the sun's ultraviolet rays full of radiation that we are supposed to avoid. Now, I was being asked to willingly submit myself to the advanced technology of smart radioactive beams, which would target and kill any micro-mutant cell that may have escaped the blitz of chemotherapy or the jaws of my protective tigers. I complied with the treatment because in 1999, thirty-three radiation treatments was the "Standard of Care" for breast cancers such as mine. However, neither mentally, nor emotionally, nor spiritually did I buy the necessity or the logic behind the treatment. I'm not saying that radiation is unnecessary. I just wasn't convinced it was necessary for me.

I was assured by my oncologist and surgeon that the chemotherapy would attack and kill my cancerous cells. But they both encouraged me to follow protocol in order to give myself all of the possible anti-cancer weapons available. My personal experience in the medical world has evolved to believe that a patient is either overtreated or undertreated. In my case, I believe radiation was overtreatment, but I did not have the guts to say, "No, thank you."

I do not ever want to look back with regret that I did not do everything possible on my own behalf. If the cancer ever returns, I want to be able to say, "I did my part."

Sometimes things remain the Standard of Care, which is a legal term. Standard of Care is the measuring stick of any medical treatment. If I have a cold, the doctor has a Standard of Care which is, "Go home, take two aspirins, and call me in the morning."

If the doctor does not follow that prescriptive Standard of Care and my cold turns into pneumonia, then I can sue him or her for not practicing a Standard of Care. That, of course, is an oversimplified explanation.

Either because of my predisposed emotional resistance to the radiation treatment, or perhaps because of just a poor personality mix, I didn't hit it off well with my radiologist. My oncologist loved my questions. My radiologist was clearly bugged by them, and was quite condescending in his answers. But by this time in treatment I was tired enough that it just didn't matter. He was here, I was here, let's get this over with.

I did not have the energy to interview another radiologist in hopes of finding a more compatible match. At the same time I was starting radiation treatment, I was also hunting for an open-minded gynecologist who was willing to grant me a hysterectomy. I was having very little success with that search and it was exhausting to keep trying. Thus, I was clearly preoccupied with that hunt and had no leftover energy to pursue a different oncology radiologist.

I continued with the radiologist I had because at least he was convenient. Radiation treatments were daily, except, of course, on weekends or holidays, where my cancer cells take the traditional work-week break. I, too, prefer not to work weekends, and prefer that my clients have their crises during the week, which some of them oblige me, and others don't. I assume that radiologists have the same agreement with cancer cells.

"Please lie dormant during the weekend."

Going daily to a fifteen minute radiation treatment was a bummer to my practice schedule which was already suffering. My clients accommodated my scheduling changes quite nicely, but the "guilty mother" part of me hated asking. The entire treatment was five and a half weeks.
I was neutral about my relationship with the radiologist and his staff until the treatments actually began. But my dislike for him and his staff crystallized during what was called the tattoo phase, which was within the first three radiation treatments. My understanding is that the job of the radiologist is to look at the x-rays of my chest, where the tumor used to be and then mathematically configure a target for the beams of radiation.

During this phase my body was manipulated this way and that way, while the treatment team marked me with blue magic markers. I was told that after a few days, when they are sure they had me positioned right, they would permanently tattoo those dots on my body. I was never asked whether that would be okay. I was never invited to participate in medical discussions about my body at all. I was, in fact, just a body lying on a cold slab of steel expected to do everything I was told to do. I happen to like tattoos and sometimes wish I had one. However, being told that my body was going to be tattooed permanently, without being invited to participate in that decision, incensed me.

CHAPTER 22

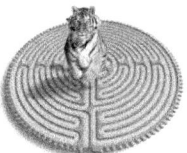

STRATEGIES FOR ASSERTIVENESS

Because I knew that there was one spot, right in the center of my neck-line, that I was unwilling to let the radiology staff tattoo, I needed to acquire some strategies for assertiveness.

Sometimes when I become that angry I cry. But this time I developed a strategy about being assertive. On the day they were supposed to tattoo my body, I said, "You may place your blue dots where you have them outlined except for this one here in the very center of my clavicle."

I was told, "No one will be able to notice these blue dots; they are small and after a time even you will forget they are there."

I kept my cool and didn't respond sarcastically with, "Excuse me, are you hearing impaired?"

I simply restated, "I said, you may go ahead and place the blue dots permanently on my body where you have them mapped except the one here."

I pointed to my throat, and to the blue magic marker dot in the very center of my neck line. "Well, I'll have to get approval from the doctor to do that," the technician said.

"Fine, do what you need to do. If the doctor has a problem with it, tell him he can talk to me. I am not going to allow either you or him to place a permanent dot where my blouse opens and where my necklaces fall. Sorry," I said with a smile.

"The doctor is not here today," he said.

I just looked at him, saying nothing. Finally, when the no-compromise look on my face convinced him that the answer was clearly and permanently no, and that in addition I was not going to rescue him by solving his problem, he said, "We can go ahead and do the treatment today and place the markers tomorrow."

I said in the friendliest, most placating voice I could drum up, "That's fine." I then walked to the table.

The next day I was told, "The doctor said, 'That's fine, we can work with the magic marker on your throat."

I wanted to say many things, but I only said, "Then fine, you may go ahead."

This is an assertiveness technique that anyone can learn and practice. I encourage you to do so. If there is anywhere in the world where excellent assertive training tools are needed, it is with the medical profession. Believe me, they are not used to you participating in your own care, making decisions on your own behalf, or challenging the decisions that they make. It takes a huge amount of patience and unrelenting assertiveness to deal with them. Assertiveness skills are required because if you get aggressive or decompensate into a bucket of tears, the medical profession will tune you out and not even try to work with you collaboratively.

Unfortunately, it is not only female psychologists who become afflicted with breast cancer. As a result, most patients don't push for what they want or need once they are stonewalled by the medical defense. This saddens me. You have a right to use your voice and to make your own medical decisions. You have the right to refuse treatment. Be advised though, when or if you ever do refuse a treatment, your doctor has a professional right, not an obligation, but a **right** to fire you from his or her practice for "non-compliance."

But if your doctor likes you, he or she will probably do what I do which is to provide a CYA note in the client's chart, "Client acted against medical advice." Then life goes on without interruption. Perhaps being fired by your doctor (not that I ever have been) is not necessarily a negative. It could be a sign that you are serious about having a voice in your medical treatment. Some doctors can't handle that. My experience tells me that those doctors who cannot handle active patient participation are not grouped by race, gender, or age. Those doctors come in all colors, ages, and genders. The good doctors also come in all colors, ages, and genders. Good and bad doctors are person-specific and not a class of people.

My radiation treatment went on without interruption. Of course, I was not emotionally connected to anyone at the radiologist's office: therefore, I never looked forward to going. I worked out a deal with my tigers where they sent me positive energy during my radiation treatment while I practiced an attitude of gratefulness. I offered prayers of gratitude for being alive and being healthy enough to withstand the Standard of Care.

I went to my thirty-three radiation treatments. They accommodated my psychotherapy practice needs at my request to have the first appointment after lunch. That appointment time guaranteed that I could be back in my office in time for my 2:00 p.m. session. At every radiation treatment, I arrived, and read a magazine until I was called. I then went to the back of the treatment room, pulled a robe off the shelf, disappeared behind a curtain, and changed. The radio was always blaring current trends in music, not anything relaxing. The technicians talked to each other as if I did not exist.

I was filled with sadness as I wrote this chapter. It makes me sad that I was so disengaged and objectified during that phase of my treatment. I know medical workers must protect themselves emotionally in order to work with a dying population, but still the industry needs to restructure how they do patient care.

Each day I was zapped with radioactive smart beams. Within a week the skin around the scar became red and itchy. Within two weeks it reddened to an irritation level. By week three, I had an ongoing burn that was comforted only at times by a radiation cream. Now, years later, my chest has a patch of discolored skin forever reminding me of the radioactive burn. The permanent blue dots are ghost-like, a haunting reminder of my past trauma.

When radiation was over, I was supposed to go back every three months for a checkup. I believe I went once, at the most twice. I saw no purpose whatsoever of returning to my radiologist to look at my chest. Dr. Langford was looking at my chest every three months in my checkups with him. I thought that would be sufficient, and thus I stopped going for radiation follow-ups. Do you think his office called? No. I was a number to them, probably one that they put in the "deceased" file.

Here again, I am not sure my insurance company appreciates the money I saved them since they keep raising my premium. But I figure I have saved them a pretty penny by not doing the radiation oncology follow-ups, not having reconstructive surgery, and not having a stem cell transplant.

Then again, insurance companies and breast cancer are perilous enemies in the pit.

CHAPTER 23

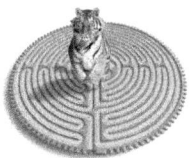

MY LOVE-HATE RELATIONSHIP WITH TAMOXIFEN

From the beginning of my dialogue with Dr. Langford, I was told, "Dr. Dilley, when you are finished with your chemotherapy you will go on a drug called Tamoxifen."

Tamoxifen has been around for thirty years and shows statistical significance against recurrences. Because my particular type of breast cancer was fed by estrogen, it was important to shut it down. Tamoxifen blocks the estrogen from my body by providing a protective shield over my estrogen receptors. As a result, estrogen cannot enter its designated receptor. Therefore, it eliminates itself from my body, just like other waste products.

However, Tamoxifen did not come without its side effects. My biggest concern was the risk of uterine cancer. It had been proven by 1999 that there was a statistical correlation between women taking Tamoxifen for breast cancer and the possibility of uterine cancer. In the next chapter you will read about my choice to have a hysterectomy, which was my response to the statistical correlation between Tamoxifen and uterine cancer. The statistics were low, only a three percent chance, but, nonetheless, a chance I was not willing to take.

I started taking the Tamoxifen concurrently with my radiation treatment. I took Tamoxifen for five years. During the radiation treatment, I tweaked my visualization a bit, picturing the radiation as tiger's breathe burning up any leftover particles of cancer cells. It was then natural to think of Tamoxifen as a "tiger pill" that would daily sit guard at the estrogen receptors.   At times, with my sense of humor, I could picture hockey games going on inside my body. The estrogen tried to make its way down the field toward the goalie. The big tiger in the goalie box used its tail to swish the estrogen hockey puck back down the court.

My relationship with Tamoxifen seemed uneventful and just part of my recovery drill. But by October 2000, I hit a wall. I could not understand what was happening to me. I looked at every angle. What had happened? How was it that I didn't care whether I got out of bed in the morning, went to work, or even took a shower for that matter?   Flicking the changer for the TV was about all I was up to. At first I thought it was the hysterectomy causing my depression. I had never before felt quite so bizarre. Images, still photo shots of bizarre thoughts, would intrude into my mind's eye. Images that were similar to Stephen King's chairs falling from the sky in his book *Hearts from Atlantis*.   I was entertained by most of my bizarre images, but did find them dreadfully distracting when trying to pay attention to my clients. It seemed like my attention span dropped to below zero. I felt agitated all of the time. I loved my job. What was going on with me?

 I spoke with my oncologist and he said, "Well, two percent of women do become depressed on the Tamoxifen."

Gee, this was a small statistic that he had failed to tell me. This time the percentage pool landed against me. Obviously, I was part of the two percent group. Clearly, this depression was chemical in nature, not situational. Thankfully, I knew enough about the shapes and sizes of depression to understand that my lack of attention, my agitation, and now extremely bizarre thoughts clearly marked a depression. However, if I had known about the two percent statistic, I might have sought psychopharmacological help before allowing the depression to become so severe.

My oncologist tried me on Prozac, which certainly was my choice and a reasonable starting medication. After a few months of Prozac, I wasn't feeling much better. My family practice physician, Dr. Birkholz, suggested Wellbutrin. It worked like a charm. I focused again, got organized, and moved paperwork off of my desk. My bizarre thinking and intrusive images went away. I finally felt normal again. My desire to work with my clients and to continue to focus on my physical healing returned.

About two months after starting the Wellbutrin I ran across an article in the psychopharmacological news that said, "Tamoxifen used to treat manic side of bipolar disorder."

I read the article, which interestingly enough had been in my in box since April 2000. I had never bothered to open it. I read with understanding, as the article articulated exactly what the Tamoxifen shuts down in the brain. So not only was it an estrogen blocker, but it also shuts down a PK6 protein that is responsible for elevated mood. No wonder I had been so flat-lined. And even on the Wellbutrin I enjoyed the ability to focus but I still was pretty flat-lined. I was finally glad to have a clear explanation of what had happened to me.

One of the reasons I am very candid about Tamoxifen is that if only two percent of the women on Tamoxifen suffer from severe depression, then something else must be going on. As a psychologist, I know that women are notorious for under-reporting symptoms so I suspect that the key to the two percent statistic is about under-reporting. However, it is also possible that two percent of us have a pre-existing anomaly with our PK6 protein. Never underestimate your intuitive side! Pay attention to how you are coping, allowing yourself to notice changes and differences that occur. Ask yourself, "What do I need to do address the difference?" Awareness and action are the keys to responsible living with breast cancer or any other disease.

It is also important to note that in 2010, new research has come to light and it is now dangerous to take an antidepressant that is a Selective Se-rotonin Reuptake Inhibitor (SSRI) while on Tamoxifen. Because this book is not intended to give any medical advice nor should it be used or interpreted as medical advice, it is important that you to stay on top of research, new data and make informed treatment choices throughout your medical journey. Be sure that you are working with an informed medical team when making difficult treatment choices, especially where one drug might be harmful to another.

Before I close this chapter about Tamoxifen, I feel it is important to say a word about weight gain and joint pain. Tamoxifen can cause a signifi-cant weight gain and by the end of my second year on the Tamoxifen, I gained twenty pounds. Nothing I did took the pounds off or reduced the numbers on the scale. The joint pain was also significant. After sit-ting for only short periods of time, I felt and looked like a very elderly lady trying to get up and move around.   My joints became tight and inflexible. These issues went away after coming off the Tamoxifen.

Needless to say neither did I like looking into the mirror and seeing a larger woman looking back at me. I understand that, in our weight conscious culture, body image and body size are a cultural ill with which we all suffer. The underlying world of the culturally-thin haunts our psyches daily with advertisements and products. I believe the mantra "thin is beautiful" bangs away at everyone's self confidence in the West-ern World.

As a psychologist, I become angry with the mentality of a skinny cul-ture. As a person gaining weight, I get frustrated with having to address the same issues my clients do regarding weight gain. However, one ad-vantage I have over them is not the fact that I am a psychologist, because that doesn't make a damn bit of difference when it comes to weight gain. I am fighting it just like everyone else right now. My advantage is that I have met and visited with my mortality personally and as a result, I am able more times than not to look at the heavier woman in the mirror and genuinely say, "Thank you for being there to look back at me."

Genuine gratitude about being alive is an experience that comes from deep inside of the "healing place," not from reading the "should be grateful" self-help books. Today, I am grateful to still be hanging out here on earth and eagerly look forward to the days ahead of me.

CHAPTER 24

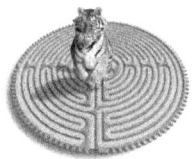

MY HYSTERECTOMY

When I finished with radiation treatment in March of 2000, I scheduled my hysterectomy for the following month. I had decided early on in my treatment that a hysterectomy would be a logical choice for me to assure myself that I would not be part of the three percent of women who get uterine cancer because of the drug Tamoxifen.

I had no idea how difficult it would be to obtain a hysterectomy from the male medical profession. Nor did I expect a fight from my insurance company. I figured with an estrogen-fed breast cancer and a three percent chance of uterine cancer that getting the insurance company to approve a hysterectomy would not be a big deal. However, even eight months of daily dealing with the medical industry didn't quite prepare me for the obstacles into which I ran.

My first visit was to a male obstetrician gynecologist (OB/GYN) to obtain my pap smear. My pap results returned with some pre-cancerous cervical cells. But this doctor did not want me to rush right into a hysterectomy. First, he wanted to observe the right protocol. He said I needed another procedure to see what the cells were doing, a procedure called a colposcopy. I knew within me that this OB/GYN was not the right doctor for me. I did not feel heard and I felt a bit placated. I believed that if I was going to get a hysterectomy, he was not my guy.

Next, I asked my oncologist for another referral. The next referral was across the Valley in northeast Scottsdale. I made an appointment with this doctor to get this second procedure done. I didn't like him much, either. He was even more condescending than the first. The colposcopy, which is a follow-up procedure to a bad pap smear, confirmed that I had dysplasia. Dysplasia is the abnormal development of immature cell growth in the cervical area. On that basis he was willing to talk to my insurance company and see if he could obtain a pre-certification for a hysterectomy; however, he informed me that usually dysplasia is not a big deal and the consensus among his colleagues and the insurance companies is usually to just keep an eye on it. By the time my results had come back, though, I was damn sure I wasn't using him. I did not like his personality and was not comfortable with him.

I still don't know why I had dysplasia. I was thankful that I had it because I hoped it would help me fit the profile for a medically necessary hysterectomy. After all, I was a breast cancer patient. Perhaps the dysplasia was caused from the chemotherapy. I normally had a Pap every two years and did not have one prior to chemotherapy. Thus, the dysplasia developed over the past two years. Perhaps my cancer was working its way into other areas of my body. It didn't really matter. I was on a mission to find someone who would help me get what I felt like I needed. Word of mouth brought me a referral, a woman by the name of Dr. Eugenie Anderson.

However, prior to meeting with this third OB/GYN, I had received so much resistance to a hysterectomy that I had asked my oncologist for a "reality check."

I asked Dr. Langford, "Am I being over-reactive here?" "Am I crazy?"

He responded, "No, Dr. Dilley, you are not crazy. There is only a three percent chance of uterine cancer with Tamoxifen, but what really matters is where you land within those statistics. If you are in the three percent, then you will have to have a hysterectomy and more radiation."

I felt validated and supported to pursue this option. I met with my Dr.

Eugenie Anderson. It was a match made in heaven. She was pleasant, warm and inviting. She also understood that a woman battling cancer wanted to be pro-active in making sure that as many as possible entry doors were shut for any cancer repeat. Her questions and concerns were genuine. I felt heard, understood, and validated. I think both of us were under the impression that obtaining a pre-certification for a hysterectomy would not be a problem. However, the first answer from the insurance company was a resounding "No."

The insurance company wanted more information. Dr. Anderson and I sat down across from each other in her office, and I answered what seemed like hundreds of other questions and we filed our appeal. Finally, an insurance review granted their omnipotent "Yes."

I entered surgery early in April and again had a complimentary one night stay in the hospital. The next day, Dr. Anderson, told me with a twinkle in her eye that the hysterectomy also confirmed that I had some endometriosis growing in my body. It was as if the twinkle in her eye was saying, "See, we proved them ,didn't we?" I felt validated.

I don't know why it was so important for me to prove the insurance company and the other two male gynecologists wrong, but it was extremely validating to me to prove them wrong. I think there is so little control we have as patients in the medical field that this battle became one of control for me. It was a win, a big win. I was doing my best to honor my intuition and do whatever it took to place as many odds on my side during this battle. Remember, you are the one in charge of your medical care. It is up to you whether you have a supportive team or not. I encourage you to keep searching; there are still good doctors out there that can hear and will respond to your needs.

CHAPTER 25

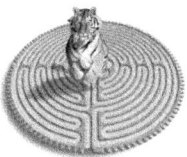

DENTISTRY AND PLACATING DOCTORS

My experience with the radiologist dogged me at my dentist's office. After I completed all of my breast cancer treatments, life returned to routine medical issues such as getting my teeth cleaned. So, on my first visit in about eighteen months my dentist's technician just automatically started preparing me for x-rays. I said to her as she placed the gray radioactive guard across my chest, "Excuse me; I am not doing x-rays today. Just clean my teeth."

"But Robin it has been almost two years since your last x-rays. We need to see if anything else is going on in there," the tech protested.

"If there is anything else going on it clearly is not bothering me. I just finished radiation treatment and I am not going to have additional radiation in my body right now," I asserted.

"Okay, we can wait until next time," she complied.

I thought, *She sure is dense. I am not having x-rays until I have a reason, such as pain. It is not like dentistry can do preventive care, except cleaning.*

It is also the Standard of Care in dental practice for the dentist to check your mouth medically after the routine teeth cleaning. The dentist entered and said, "Robin, I understand you didn't want x-rays because of your radiation treatment. The radiation I use here is no different than being out in the sun for fifteen minutes or so."

"I understand the radiation for x-rays may not seem that significant to you. However, I do notice that each time you take x-rays I am always cloaked in a gray radiation shield. I don't usually wear something like that if I am going out into the sun. And besides, my radiologist told me never to be in the full sun even with sunscreen. He told me if I swam in the middle of the day or went to the beach, to please wear at least a white t-shirt rather than have my radiated area directly exposed to the sun."

The dentist said nothing. He just began searching my mouth with his pick instruments. I mean, what could he say about the radiation shield they put around me? Nothing! I had beaten him at his own game. I had prevailed concerning my desires, and that was that.

I believe I went back to that dentist twice after that experience for routine cleaning. Each time it was a fight over the radiation. Each time I received the same placating, "No different than being out in the sun." He also reminded me that I had a tooth that needed work according to past x-rays.

When I found a new dentist, he manually looked at all of my teeth with his tools for poking and prodding. No previous dental problems were discovered that needed correction. It was during this experience with the new dentist that I reached the conclusion that perhaps my former dentist was more interested in the gold lining his pockets than my need to feel safe. Currently, I obtain my dental work in Mexico.

Once again, I don't want to sound preachy, but your health care is **your** health care. Therefore, you are the one responsible for it, allowing or not allowing decisions to be made about you and your body. The final responsibility is in your court. If you stay involved and pro-active, you will feel less of a victim in this world of medical practice. The operative word is "practice."

I understand what practice means, owning my own psychotherapy practice. Each day I am dumbstruck by the magical and mystical soul that responds differently to different interventions and acts of empathy. Each client is different. My interventions with one client cannot be patented to provide the same outcome to another client. I have to be on my toes, awake, alert, watching for the window of opportunity to make my move as a psychotherapist. When that move is in sync with the client, awesome things happen in my office. When I push too hard, hold back, or become bored, something is off-kilter and it is my job to figure out what it is and adjust to what is happening in the session.

I find that if I allow myself to keep the word "practice" in the foreground it makes me a much better listener. I remain humble knowing I am blessed with a gift and I must use it with tenderness and academic accuracy.

Placating doctors and other bothersome folks is a well-documented theory in the field of psychotherapy. Placating is one of the four types of dysfunctional communication styles that Virginia Satir, the world renowned family therapist, talked about in her book *The New People Making*. According to Satir, there are four universal patterns of communication styles that people use to conceal feelings of weakness, low self-esteem or threat. These four patterns are blaming, computing, distracting or placating.

Blaming, of course, is that of fault-finding, causing others to feel inferior. Computing is the act of being very correct, very reasonable, showing no feeling, which is the type of communication often replicated in the medical field. Distractions within communication are those actions that are irrelevant to what anyone else is saying or doing. For me, placating communication is the worst type of dysfunctional communication. I react strongly when I think the people are using placating forms of communication with me. I think they believe I am stupid. I suspected that the dialogue in my dentist's head was something like, "The poor darling doesn't understand that these dental x-rays are absolutely harmless."

It was placating communication that I thought the radiologist used with me. I always have lots of questions for Dr. Langford. Dr. Langford seems to appreciate my questions and research. I was validated by being an active participant in my process, but the radiologist seemed to be bothered by my active participation. Somehow, it felt as if I was slowing him down, getting in his way. I find it interesting that I am not disclosing his name, not because I choose to protect my experience of him from him or others, but because I truly do not remember his name. And, as dismissive as he was to me it is now my turn to be dismissive. Searching for his name is not worth the time it takes to check my medical records.

The point of all of my communication about placating doctors is to help demonstrate to you how important I feel it is for you to feel respected, safe, and comfortable with your medical team and the lifesaving decisions you have to make on your behalf. It is important that you feel mutual respect for and from your medical team. It is impossible for you to like everyone and for everyone to like you. That is an old Rational Emotive Therapy truism, a la Albert Ellis (the father of this therapeutic approach). We are socialized to want people to like us. We are taught as children to adapt our behavior in ways that please other people. Thus, when we are vulnerable and needy we are trained to do as we are told to keep everyone happy – and heaven forbid tick off the doctor treating you. Albert Ellis teaches his clients to give up the ideal that everyone is going to like you. Not everyone is going to like you, and matter of fact some people may actually hate you versus just being neutral about you.

With health care being what it is currently in the United States, it is still important to choose a treatment team that you believe in and that you enjoy seeing.   When you are having to spend more time than it takes getting a prescription for your allergies with a person in the medical field, I believe it is important that you are fond of that person and that you have a sense they respect you and the difficult choices you are having to make. Please remember, it is okay to be the captain of your own team, and if you do not believe you have the expertise to do that, then choose someone you trust and believe in to help facilitate this difficult medical process with you.

CHAPTER 26

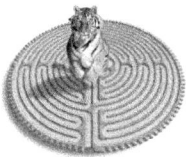

BREAST CANCER AND INSURANCE COMPANIES

As a clinical psychologist, I had a pre-existing condition before I began dealing with my health insurance. My pre-existing condition was called "intense dislike" for all health insurance companies. Up until January 2010, there was no parity for psychologists. Parity means that insurance companies must pay the same percentage to psychologists for mental health coverage as they pay for a primary care doctor visit. Without parity insurance companies pick and choose what they pay mental health providers. What that has meant is that if you have 80/20 plan for your medical coverage, then if you are seeing an MD for a cold, your insurance company will pay eighty percent of the MD's fee. However, if you are suffering from a depressive or anxiety disorder, your health insurance company pulls down a bogus number from the air and may only pay fifty percent of seventy dollars. If mental health providers had parity, then the insurance company would have to do something honorable and pay eighty percent of our usual and customary fee which in Arizona is anywhere from $125 to $250 per session hour. Supposedly parity was enacted as law in 2010, but I am not sure about that because I do not take health insurance. My clients must bill their own insurance companies. I understand that is a clear inconvenience especially to someone who is already depressed, but my counter-transference has not proven healthy for my professional relationship with my clientele. Counter-transference is a therapeutic term that means that I as the therapist am having an emotional reaction to my client that is hindering my therapeutic judgment.

After dealing with my own health care insurance company over the past ten years, I have upgraded my pre-existing condition from "intense dislike" to "intense disgust."   Until our nation does something to correct the inequity of health care in America, we are all victims of insurance companies, especially those unfortunates that have to deal with managed care systems or HMO plans. The new health care reform bill was passed before the publishing of this book, and I really do not understand the hatred that it has stirred.   However, that is a different topic for a different time.

I was prepared to have nothing but a hassle from my insurance company. However, I was pleasantly surprised that throughout my treatment they paid for everything willingly, without a fight, except for the fight over my hysterectomy. They were even willing to pay for my stem cell transplant, had I chosen to go that direction. While I was considering the stem cell transplant, they assigned to me my own personal case manager to facilitate answering any questions. However, after discussing the stem-cell transplant with the case manager, it appeared I had completed more hours of research on the subject than the case manager and that I had a better understanding of the pros and cons of the treatment.   It was still satisfying to know that I was being provided with an advocate had I needed one. Until we talked, he was unaware that the results of stem cell transplants for stage two breast cancer were not statistically significant when compared to the treatment ascribed to the traditional Standard of Care.

I do not readily have the financial figures that my breast cancer cost my insurance company. Neither do I know to the penny how much money I saved them. I do know that they saved close to a $100,000 when I declined the stem cell transplant and an additional $40,000 when I declined reconstructive surgery. Even though I advocated for a hysterectomy that they eventually paid for, I saved them additional thousands of dollars not to have to treat uterine cancer had I been one of those unlucky ones in the three percent pool of Tamoxifen caused uterine cancer. I sang praises about my insurance company throughout my treatment.

What I didn't know at the time was that when the next renewal date rolled around that my insurance premiums would triple. I was irate when I read my new statement. I just couldn't believe the jump. My premiums went from $104 a month to $312 a month. What a shock. I would have thought tripling my premium like that would be illegal, but it wasn't illegal for them to do this. The following year the monthly premium went up to $402. I finally changed my deductible to lower my monthly cost. Five years post-treatment I paid a $1,500 dollar deductible and a $497 monthly premium. In 2008, I was paying $876 a month for my premium, plus a $3,000 deductible. I cried "uncle" in 2009, and went to a $5,000 deductible and a $565 a month premium. One year later they increased it another $100 to $675 a month. I am not eligible to change insurance companies because with a diagnosis of breast cancer, nobody wants me. I can't even qualify for long-term health insurance because I had more than four lymph nodes involved in the cancer. Thankfully, I had disability insurance prior to my breast cancer diagnosis. Hopefully I will never need it.

I found disparate numbers on breast cancer costs when I went to the World Wide Web, to check out how much a typical stage two breast cancer costs insurance companies to treat it. As a result, I chose not to make this chapter a treatise on the cost, but a reminder to you that, whether or not your insurance company likes it, you do have some rights. Be a wise consumer, find out what your rights are and force your insurance company to comply with those rights.

Insurance companies can be rather patronizing and placating too. It seems they don't think patients have brains. They don't believe we can figure out what is best for us in the long run. If insurance companies chose to be more collaborative and less defensive, and more prevention-orientated and less disease-focused, then the United States would be a much happier place when it comes to health care. I am positive that anyone who has had a major medical problem has their own insurance story to tell. Perhaps the _Chicken Soup for the Soul_ series, that multitude of books by Jack Canfield, should offer a book on *Recovering from Your Insurance Trauma: Stories of Woe and Despair, Moving Toward Victory and Resolution*.

After my long journey and challenges with insurance companies, I would like to share with you some of what I have learned with the hope of reducing the unneeded stress in your life.

Helpful Suggestions for Dealing with Your Insurance Company

KNOW YOUR RIGHTS...

- Read the fine print of your policy from cover to cover. Use a magic marker to highlight areas that you are concerned about.

- Ask for clarification on those areas.

- Seek legal counsel if you have concerns or questions about the language and do not feel you are getting the "REAL ANSWER" to your question.

- When you call, document the name of the person you talk to, including the date and time.

- Ask that person to fax you that information in writing. (They usually will not, but ask and document their response.)

- Remember, you are the consumer, and you pay their salary. Start off your conversation in a tone that is optimistic, kind, and gentle. Remember, the person you are speaking with did not write the policy. And they are probably stuck with the same bad insurance you have.

- Ask for a supervisor if you are not happy.

- Call your insurance agent if you need to enlist help.

- Call and write your state insurance commissioner to report unfair treatment.

- Do not hesitate to ask for the medical treatment that you and your doctor think would be best for you. If it is not in their system, they still have to provide it for you because it is now "medically necessary." Insist on your rights.

Here are a couple of other thoughts that you might find helpful.

Here in this state, local news stations are always looking for unfair stories to air on the prime-time news hour. Ordinary citizens like you and I can call most stations and have the unfairness of any situation aired on prime-time. Just the threat of calling the news station is enough to obtain a different and positive response.

Also, a note about research: In the medical field treatments and standards of care change overnight. For instance, at the time of my treatment PET Scans were new. As a result the procedure needed to be pre-certified by my insurance company. Usually the first answer out of the insurance company's mouth is "NO." Thus, when my blood work was elevated Dr. Langford liked to follow up with a PET scan. My first PET scan was in 2002. My insurance company fought paying for my first PET scan in December 2002. But after an appeal, they had to pay. On the PET scan that I received in the spring of 2004, my insurance company didn't even need to pre-certify it, because now PET scans have become the Standard of Care for appropriately diagnosing breast cancer. PET scans now offer cost-effective and diagnostic accuracy in treating cancers. If you are having a difficult time getting your insurance company to pay for a treatment because it is new, keep appealing. Also, check to see if Medicare is paying for the procedure. If Medicare pays for a procedure that means Medicare has accepted the procedure as a Standard of Care. Once Medicare approves any treatment all insurance companies must follow suit. To find out more information and current statistics on PET scan treatment, go to www.breastcancer.org.

CHAPTER 27

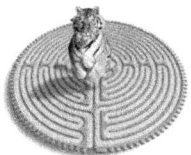

DOING THE NOW

Breast cancer provides me with a mantra that I call "doing the now." It is there as my constant reminder that today, this moment is the only one I have, so I must make the most of it, enjoy it, and make it count, because in a moment's notice it can all go away. From this space inside of me, I challenge myself to take risks that I know I never would have taken without breast cancer egging me on. I would have allowed my shyness, awkwardness, or negative self talk to get in my way, limiting my desires and dreams. I do believe that in order to take risks, we must get out of our box and certainly out of our comfort zone.

I was presented with an opportunity of risk-taking in the fall of 2000. The Phoenix Mercury, our Women's National Basketball Association (WNBA) franchise, was hosting a "Fantasy Camp." The purple flyer read, "Treat yourself to a once in a lifetime opportunity. Come play basketball with the professionals Jennifer Gillom, Lisa Harrison, Tonya Edwards and Michelle Cleary."

I blushed just reading it. My heart leapt at the opportunity but my mind clamped down like a crushing device, shutting off any minuscule hope that I would be foolish enough to play with the real players. The shrieking, shaming clamor echoed in my head of, *Oh no, I can't do that. I can't even dribble the ball up and down the court, much less box out in a defensive position. Who am I trying to fool?*

Pam picked up a copy of the same flyer and said, "Why don't you go? I will treat you for your birthday."

My birthday was in October; the camp was actually on my birthday weekend. I said, "No I can't do that. I am too shy, too old, and not good enough to play."

Pam replied, "It is a fantasy camp. It is about your fantasy – not about your ability to play basketball."

"I'll think about it," I said.

And I did. Each time I pictured myself showing up and dribbling the ball down the court, I felt queasy in my stomach and I flushed with color. But I had pledged that now I would allow nothing to stand in my way of doing the things I wanted to do. I graciously accepted Pam's gift and went off to play with the big girls.

What a hoot! I knew I was using breast cancer as my teacher. It felt good to challenge myself in that way. It makes me sad that I had to lean on something like breast cancer to help me take certain risks. However, I know that is true for so many of us.

I, like most people, often live in my head, only imagining what life could be like with the wishes, should've, could've, would've – but never venturing beyond my emotional limitations to live my dreams. I hate that it took cancer to make me challenge myself to live my life more fully. But cancer had a way of screaming in my face, "Now or never – you choose!"

I knew that I could still give in to feelings of shyness and intimidation, and that I didn't have to allow breast cancer to be my teacher. I could've chosen to resent it, be depressed, or angry over it. Thankfully, I have not allowed myself to do that. I might be terrified or overly cautious about having breast cancer, but thankfully I was not resentful or angry about it. Things happen and breast cancer is one of those things that happened to me and thousands of other women and men. (Yes, men do get breast cancer.)

I knew I had to get through cancer the best way I knew how. Taking the path of least resistance, I chose to accept it and embraced it for its teaching while I defined positive ways to make myself as healthy as possible both physically and emotionally. As a result, I have played, traveled, and written – things that I would not have taken the time to do before breast cancer.

CHAPTER 28

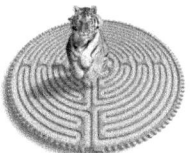

FANTASY CAMP

The Mercury Fantasy Camp was three full days of drills, games, and physical endurance. Each morning was packed with constant action and pleasant encouragement from that team of four, Cleary, Edwards, Gillom and Harrison. All of us fantasy players enjoyed learning how to box out, follow through and even use the often performed pick and roll. From my point of view, everyone seemed to enjoy being there, including the team of four.

We developed camaraderie and mutual respect for each other. Each fantasy member had a different reason to be there. I was no longer bald, so I could share or not share why I had chosen to attend. With some I did, with others I chose not to share my story.

Each afternoon, we were divided up into teams and played each other, with a championship game taking place on the third day.

The camp made me aware of how out of shape and stiff I had become over the years. But more importantly, I became even more aware of my inner space that filled daily with powerful emotions like joy, delight, and a sense of accomplishment. For me, the Fantasy Camp was more about overcoming my shyness than learning basketball moves. I didn't have a lot of eye-hand coordination as a child. Since I became an adult, it certainly has improved some, but slight improvement did not help me master dribbling the ball around my body and through my legs.

There are as many ways to package and play basketball as there are to package and tackle mental health issues. Here are four keys of positive mental health that I have tried to practice over the years.

Key #1. *Make sure that you practice excellent self-care emotionally, physically, intellectually, and spiritually.*

Key #2. *Remain fluid and flexible, maintaining a stance of unconditional positive regard for yourself and others.*

Key #3. *Maintain the ability to take risks and play hard. Look for opportunities to get ahead of the game.*

Key #4.   *Follow your heart. That is where your dreams are.*

So paying homage to these four keys, I felt compelled to practice what I preached. All things considered, I did pretty well during the Fantasy Camp.

The camp also allowed me opportunity to reflect on an article I wrote in my 1999 BETWEEN THE SPACES: HEALING FOR OUR LIVES newsletter. Just as I was being diagnosed with breast cancer a WNBA player, Kim Perrot, was dying of lung cancer.

I have provided an excerpt here. I wrote:

Kim Perrot of the Houston Comets died from lung cancer before the season was over. Kim provided the fans with an opportunity to watch her play with passion, drive and enthusiasm Kim was a walk-on, meaning she went down to Houston's gym and worked out with the team in hopes of gaining a spot on the team. Everyone wanted Kim to be successful. If she were successful, it meant that other women who didn't make it to the WNBA draft could also have hope. Any player's success is our success as women.

When Kim Perrot died, it was hard and unsettling to many people and players that knew her so well. For me, a certain somberness settled in my soul that pointed out to me that not everyone survives when they are diagnosed with cancer.

A few years after Fantasy Camp, one of the camp members by the name of Stormy was diagnosed with lung cancer, which eventually took her life but never her spirit. There seems to be certain solidarity among women with cancer, regardless of what type. Being a Survivor only heightens my prior commitment to life. And the gift of the scar and tightness in my chest is a daily reminder that today is mine and what I do with it is the result of my choices. Mortality becomes a constant friend sitting on my shoulder and coaching me through the day. The Mercury Fantasy Basketball Camp allowed me to challenge myself, push my limits, fight my shyness, and be ever-present to enjoy the moment. It was awesome. It is an experience that I recommend to anyone who loves basketball.

I returned to the Fantasy Camp in 2001. There was no such program for 2002. I believe one reason that Fantasy Camp didn't continue is because even though there may be thousands of women in the WNBA stands who would love to go to Fantasy Camp, it takes an abundance of courage. It is very hard to muster up enough courage to go mingle with athletes who box out and shoot three pointers for a living.

A Priceless Birthday Gift.

Before I conclude this chapter, I want to share with you another first and perhaps an even more amazing exploit than Fantasy Camp. Without my knowledge, Pam bid on the WNBA on-line auction for Breast Health Awareness in November of 2002. Pam won a game of HORSE with Jennifer Gillom for my 48th birthday. It is difficult for me to explain what it feels like to have a successful WNBA player come to an undisclosed location and play a game of HORSE one on one with me. The game of HORSE was around when I was a kid and maybe years before then. Just in case you have never heard of this game, this is how

I played with Jennifer. The goal is to be the last person to collect all of the letters spelling HORSE. Player #1 shoots the ball from any position around the basket. If Player #1 makes the shot, Player #2 must shoot the ball from the same position. If player #2 misses, then player #2 gets the letter H. If player #2 makes the same shot as player #1, then player #2 gets to shoot from any position around the court and Player #1 must follow. The ball goes back and forth until one player has all of the letters in HORSE. The other person wins the game. Jennifer was gracious enough to let me start but needless to say it was a very short game, so we played several.

 I will never forget the feeling of that day, the smell of threatening rain in the air, Jennifer's gentle smile, and the power of connection that saturated the grey, misty afternoon. There was no doubt that I was loved by my partner Pam, and no doubt that Jennifer Gillom genuinely cared about the cause of breast cancer and about her WNBA fans.

Let me invite you to think about the things you have missed in your life that you wanted to do, because you were too shy or uncomfortable, and ask yourself, "If I was given notice today that I had six months to live, would I take this opportunity?" That question will help you to decide whether or not it is something you really have a passion to do or if it is just a fleeting thought.

CHAPTER 29

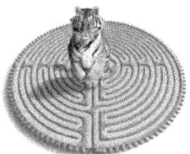

THE IMPACT OF BREAST CANCER ON RELATIONSHIPS

Perhaps my life partner Pam should have written this chapter. She tells me that she felt like she was going to pass out as she stood by my hospital bed in the recovery room when they told me I had breast cancer. I said the nasty little four letter word that begins with an "f". (There are few appropriate times to use that word, and for me that was one of them.) I had nothing for her. In that moment it was about me and there was no one for Pam.

Pam reports that she felt her knees buckle and she held onto the bed rail. I imagine it was desperately lonely for her to go home that night without me, and that each time I held my breath she held hers twice as long.

Let's face it. If I die, I am done. She is left with all of the arrangements and the chore of taking care of what I have left behind, but most of all, she is left. Her life changes forever, but her life continues. Who knows about mine?

It is a solitary experience to be the partner of a person who has a chronic or acute illness. Pretending day after day, going on as if life is normal when the relationship has been handed a "Your Time Might be Running Out" notice doesn't work very well. You must learn to talk about the illness together. You must find ways in the relationship to discuss medical treatment and worst case scenarios. You must never give up on dreaming and planning the future as if you are going to live forever. Finding that balance as you consider the possibilities of both living and dying sways you back and forth as if one minute you are performing a powerful ballet and the next minute moving to the intensity of a salsa number.

For me, Pam did an excellent job of pacing me, allowing me my deep quiet time where I cocooned and did not talk about it. She also invited me to talk about it if I wanted to. She let me know when she needed to talk about it. We were able to discuss our fears with each other, but not allow our fears to become a burden to each other. She placed no demands on me, and even suggested I take disability and stay home during the process. But when she understood how important it was for me to keep my life as normal as possible, she honored my request.

The impact of a serious illness on a relationship is real. If a relationship is already rocky, the stress on the relationship caused by an illness may become overpowering. As a psychologist, I know that this type of illness or any stressful situation taxes a relationship and can create its own separate set of problems. Sometimes fighting, addictions, and other issues escalate in order to distract from the fear and loneliness of the present. Doctors' appointments inundate your days, bills come for every piece of cotton swab you use, and the stress of feeling tired, achy, and lethargic eats away at the structure of the relationship. The familiar between the two of you becomes unfamiliar. You may find yourself wondering if there ever was a life before cancer. Being limited and not being able to do some of the simplest things, like walk up a staircase without labored breathing, become daily reminders that an invader has entered the relationship, clearly uninvited.

Pam and I live our relationship in conventional and non-conventional ways. We were aware entering this journey that this would be stressful and chose to discuss the things that made us afraid, mad or lonely. We also were aware that being in a non-conventional same sex relationship might play its way out in unusual ways in the medical field. In the beginning, Pam offered to be only introduced as my "friend." However, I am who I am and having a secret would have added additional stress to the relationship, and perhaps to making medical decisions. So from the beginning she was introduced as my partner. On paperwork when asked about "Are you in a relationship?" I always answer in the other column, "domestic partner." I felt no need to either change that or explain it in this situation. I am pleased to report that not once did our sexual orientation or domestic partnership become an obstacle.

Many times throughout this journey I was asked what to do, what to expect, by partners of friends, clients and colleagues, each of whom had just found out that a significant other was diagnosed with cancer of one kind or another. Each time I told them that it is a very personal journey for each couple. The key to every relationship is the quality of the communication.

Partners of cancer patients can have a very hard time. I cannot imagine that there is a lonelier position to be in life. You are in a very powerless place. When humans are rendered powerless, all of our defense mechanisms kick in as we try desperately to find a place of emotional safety again. These defensive reactions can look like various things in a relationship. It can feel like abandonment, and some partners leave their partners/patients because they simply cannot face losing them one step at a time. Other people become controlling, micro-managing every food, drink, and environmental suspect that their partners come in contact with, unconsciously seeking a way to control the uncontrollable.

What is helpful is to be supportive and not afraid. That is neither easy nor simple to pull off when you are feeling terrified of losing your life partner and are overpowered with helpless feelings. Helplessness, I believe, is the hardest part of the journey for everyone. However, the patient has at least the illusion of being able to take an active role in the treatment by being the recipient of chemo, radiation and surgical procedures.

As the partner of someone with breast cancer, you may feel like you have to watch helplessly, because you are not able to "fix it." There are some things you can do that might be helpful to your partner; however, it is probably advisable for you and your partner to figure out what works best through honest communication with each other. Talk together about how to proceed. The reality is that if you had a poor communication pattern before cancer, cancer certainly is not going to fix the communication pattern. Thus, a cancer diagnosis presents a compelling reason to seek out a psychologist or mental health professional to help the two of you work through difficult conversations.

Below are some suggestions for the spouses, partners, friends and family members of those with chronic or acute illnesses.

(1.) Make sure you have a support system separate from your partner to talk things through, especially yours fears and perhaps your frustration with your partner during some of this journey. You may think your partner can do more than she/he is doing to fight the cancer. You might wish she/he would make different treatment decision than she/he is making. You might be squeamish around blood or medical procedures and vomit. You will need your own support system. You cannot be her/his only support system, either. If you live in a bigger city such as Los Angeles, Phoenix, or New York, you will find numerous resources for you and your partner. In smaller cities, support systems are not so easy to find. It is possible that you may have to go to a chronic illness support group or church prayer group to receive some external support. Regardless of where you live, you may be able to connect with an online support group on the Internet.

(2.) As a partner, you will probably find that this process is also your journey, and that you are changed by it. You may discover that you are more courageous, confident and capable than you ever thought possible. Embrace these positive changes. Don't infringe on your partner's need to handle things the way she/he needs to handle them. Her/his survival drive has kicked in and nothing else matters to her/him at this point except surviving. However, each person chooses to survive in her/his own way; some of those choices are conscious and others are subconscious. Your partner may become very different than how you have known her/him to be in the past; she/he may even feel like a stranger to her/himself. You may become a stranger to yourself as well. You may discover that you are crying at the drop of a hat, becoming angry or hurt at things that would have never bothered you in the past.

(3.) I would suggest that you search for recommendations for a professional mental health provider that can help you with this difficult time. From a personal perspective, I do not believe that psychotherapist has to be a cancer survivor. In the beginning of my journey, someone else's cancer was more than I could or wanted to handle. When you are asking for referrals, the best place to start is with your primary care provider or friends and family members. A good therapist is a good therapist regardless of the issues. A bad therapist is a bad therapist regardless of the issues. That is my personal and my professional opinion. I do believe that specialists are necessary for some things such as personality disorders and serious mental illness. I also believe that children need expert mental health professionals trained specifically to treat children.

But when it comes to the human condition of living or dying, a therapist that comes with a good recommendation is the perfect place to start. THERE IS NO SHAME IN HAVING A PERSONAL THERAPIST. I BELIEVE EVERYONE SHOULD HAVE ONE. LIFE IS HARD. It is good to have someone on board in case things get really rocky, or the outcome is not what you had hoped for. At least by that time you will have a positive therapeutic relationship established with someone, rather than trying to establish one in the middle of chaos and emotional turmoil.

(4.) I believe it is helpful to your partner if they do not to have to worry about you during this time, so please find helpful ways to practice good self-care. Your life must go on, and you must not lose touch with all of the elements of your normal existence, such as work, other friendships, and personal interests. Self-care is the best gift of all that you can give your partner. Self-care is different for each person, but each of you must be able to do things that help you feel good about your choices. It may be as simple as going to movie, local coffee shop, or taking a trip down the aisles of a library or museum just to get away for a bit and distract yourself from the constant nagging fear that is going on in the background of your mind. Your partner with breast cancer may need to rent movies and indulge in a movie marathon. Positive distraction will be good for both of you. One of the things that I don't think I mentioned directly is that chemotherapy will compromise the immune system. So for at least the first nine days after a chemo treatment, your partner will need to stay away from situations that might expose her/him to other people's sicknesses. Going to a movie theater or attending a play is okay some of the time, but environmental issues and potential health hazards must be taken into consideration. All chemotherapy patients are highly susceptible to any infection or airborne virus due to their compromised immune system.

(5.) One of the most important activities that I appreciated my partner doing with me was her sitting with me as I read hundreds of pages of Internet information, and perused the pages of Susan Love's technical descriptions. I also enjoyed the times when she found articles and gave me other information that I could either choose or not choose to read at the time. It really helped me not to feel so lonely. It is a solitary journey for both of you, any way you look at it. The more support both of you have the better, but a support system of a thousand cannot take away the entire pit of loneliness in the innermost parts of your beings during this frightening time. But it can sure help.

CHAPTER 30

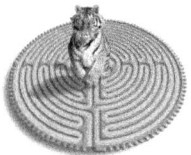

THE SEA OF PINK; A BIG SUPPORT SYSTEM

In the United States, the name Susan G. Komen (SGK) and the words breast cancer are almost synonymous. However, until you actually experience a race from the inside out, it is impossible to comprehend the emotion that can overwhelm you. For me it is an intense emotional journey that continues from the time I pick up my pink shirt until the closing celebration. The runner's finish line is not the end of the event. After the walk/race event there is a huge closing celebration, where hundreds of women just like me march into the closing ceremony with pink carnations carrying signs that represent their number of years of survivorship!

I believe the first Susan G. Komen Race in Phoenix was in 1992. At that time, I was working with a client who was diagnosed with breast cancer during her psychotherapy process. During the Eighties and Nineties, I participated in fun runs in order to collect t-shirts and free vendor items, as well as to enjoy the excitement of being with a group of adults competing to just finish a three or six-mile run. I realize that every community may not have fun-runs but here in Arizona there are lots of them and they are a major money-maker for almost any cause. I don't remember much about my first SGK run, except for the request to wear the names of the person you were running for on the back of your shirt. My shirt was white. Those who had breast cancer wore pink shirts. At that time I had only one name, the name of my client. It never crossed my mind that in just another seven years I would be wearing a pink shirt with my own name on my back.

Thus, in October of 1999, completely bald, I participated in my first SGK race wearing a pink shirt. I had no idea as to what to expect and I certainly was not prepared to see the parade of cars searching for parking spaces, nor the sea of peoples' faces wearing pink shirts. It was an overwhelming emotional experience, and one that I am not sure I can actually articulate.

Women, men, and children kept streaming out of parking garages and onto the square where tents full of vendors were giving away free goodies. I felt a sense of solidarity and purpose. I did notice I was not making much eye contact with people and was sort of sneaking glances to see how many pink shirts were around me. I am sure that for every pink-shirted participant, there were two or three supporters running with her or him, but the pink was almost blinding.

Next I saw the sign "Survivors Tent." I did not want to go there. I thought -- certainly there must have been a mistake. I was certain that if I looked down, my shirt would be white. I thought, *Can I wake up now?* At the survivor's tent I received a "goody bag" with special things like a key chain, kerchief, and various other pink items. Along with the goody bag, I received my first pink hat and white round sticker to write the number that represented the years I had been a survivor. My hat said two months. There was also a survivor breakfast for us. At that time I did not want to eat with other pink-shirted people. We were directed to tables where we found white bibs of paper and black felt pens to write the names of the people we wanted to represent. We wrote the names of the survivors that we were running for on a white bib that said "In Celebration Of." And if race participants were running for those who have died from breast cancer they wrote the names on a different bib that said "In Memory Of." That year I had no "In Memory Of" names on my bib. I only had four names on my survivor bib. Now, eleven years later. there is hardly room for all of the names on the "In Celebration Of" bib and the "In Memory Of" bib is a list of many people who have crossed my path since then. At my first race, I fought tears all morning and, eleven years later, I still wrestle with tears at the race.

CHAPTER 31

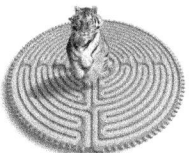

KIM'S STORY

Breast cancer has a way of connecting people in very intimate ways. It brings new people into your life while it builds bridges of re-connection to those people who have crossed your path in times past. I believe breast cancer creates an immediate bond and intimacy between souls.

In my field, the word "intimacy" is used to denote a depth, a vulnerability, a personal nakedness and trust that is sometimes extremely difficult to obtain and maintain in a relationship. Because the words "breast cancer" can reduce a person to helplessness in a matter of seconds, intimacy is constantly knocking at our door. We can either defend against it, making vain attempts to block it out, or we can gently invite it into our innermost being.

Kim and I reconnected as a result of our breast cancer. When I first met Kim, I was her instructor at Ottawa University, where I was an adjunct faculty. Ottawa caters to adults returning to college; therefore, I estimated that Kim was in her thirties. Later, I discovered we were the same age. Kim was a very bright and engaging student. I can still see exactly where she sat, with her beautiful smile and long flowing hair, and remember clearly the intensity she displayed about learning. "Inquisitive" and "zestful" are two words I used to describe her.

The other day, I found a letter I had written for Kim's internship. I wrote, *"It is clear that Kim is an asset to the programs at Parents Anonymous, not only in the services she contributes, but also in the way in which she provides vision and optimism to the organization."*

That is how I viewed Kim. She was cheerful and positive, a delight to be around. Kim graduated and went on to live her life. I wondered from time to time what had happened to Kim.

On October 13, 2000, I participated in my second Susan G. Komen Race for the Cure. My hair had grown back and I was finished with all of my treatments except for Tamoxifen and three-month checkups. Driving to the race, I felt the sense of enthusiasm in the air. As we approached the sign that flashed "event parking," other cars appeared from the morning darkness and the crowds began to take shape. A chill ran down my spine as I stepped out of the truck and into the sea of pink shirts, many of them outfitted with bibs of paper penned with the messages "In Memory Of" and "In Celebration Of." I breathed a thank-you to God.

The chill hounded me all morning. From the time I put on my pink survivor shirt and my race number to when I ran through the Tunnel of Hope, the chill would rise up in my throat, sting my eyes, and I would send it back to that dark inner chamber. For some reason, it felt like a day preplanned by a source greater than myself.

After the race, Pam, some friends, and I were standing around talking. Before any of us realized it, a Channel 12 news reporter poked a microphone into our circle and began to ask questions. "Why are you here?" "Why do you run this race?" And then the mike pointed directly to me, "Why is your shirt different from your friends' here?"

 The chill swept over me and I babbled out something. I have a hard time speaking about close emotional issues without tears coming along for the ride. For whatever reason, Channel 12 chose to show that five-second clip of me on the news that evening. I received calls that night from friends saying, "saw you both on television."

The next day when I checked my voice mail, I heard, "Robin, this is Kim. I was a student in your classes at Ottawa. You may not remember me, it has been so long."

Her voice was breaking when she added, "I think I saw you on the news last night. I am not sure it was you, but it sure looked like you. I don't know why you were on – if you were just participating in the race or if you have breast cancer. If you don't mind, will you call me? I am living in North Central Arizona near Lake Powell in a small town called Page. I was diagnosed in April with stage four breast cancer. I wanted to thank you for running in the race for whatever reason. If you have breast cancer, I would love to talk to you, talk to someone who has been there."

As I hung up the phone from that voice message, I stared off into space while that familiar chill permeated my whole body. I saw my next two clients while I was trying to get up enough courage to return Kim's call. It was seeping into my consciousness that I now knew two students, who were both going to die with this disease. Even though I know breast cancer is not contagious, there was something foreboding about being with someone who I knew was going to die. Kim's call had also brought front and center my own mortality again. *Will I be next?* echoed deep inside of my dark space. I called her back and she told me her horror story.

"Robin? Thanks so much for calling. How are you? Do you remember me?"

"Yes, Kim, I remember you. You took the classes Suicide Syndrome and Family System Techniques from me. Then I did your supervision for your internship at Parents Anonymous. You loved to run and during class coffee breaks we talked about shin splints and our latest runs."

"I saw you on Channel 12. Do you have breast cancer, too?" Kim asked.

"I am so surprised you saw me on the news, but thankful. Yes, Kim, I was diagnosed in August 1999."

"What kind?" she asked.

"Stage two, estrogen positive, aggressive," I responded.

"Oh, Robin, I am so sorry. It is awful, isn't it?"

"Yes, Kim, it's awful and scary. Tell me about you. You said on your message you were diagnosed this past April with stage four. I am sorry to hear that!" I kept my tone even and the chill at bay.

"It has been a very long ride. I started having problems over a year ago. I ached. You know me. I thought it was because I wasn't active enough and so I increased my exercise. I put on a lot of weight with no apparent reason. My hip became so painful that I dragged my leg along behind me. I kept saying I am too young for anything to be wrong. Then I began to have some problems with my implants and thought that they were probably leaking and that is why I was tired. Robin, I had to fight them to remove the implants. They kept telling me it wasn't the implants, nothing was wrong. But finally after months of fighting, I won and they scheduled to remove them. What a surprise. I had a local anesthetic and was awake when I heard the doctor say, 'What is wrong here? What is this stuff?'

"They went in to remove the implants and underneath I was full of breast cancer. Poor John was outside waiting for what was supposed to be a fairly short procedure. When the doctor came out an hour after he was supposed to, he told John, 'The implant was embedded in rock hard tissue that appears to be cancer and we had to chisel it out.'"

Kim went on, "Robin, The cancer was everywhere under the implants. They removed as much as they could. Then when I had my bone and

CT scan they discovered that cancer was all throughout my bones. That was the problem with my hip. It was full of cancer. My breast cancer is stage four and is called inflammatory breast cancer."

Kim had already explained the stage four diagnosis when she left her message on my voice mail. I knew I was not going to be hearing a positive story, but I was not quite prepared for the rest of her story. I said, "Kim, I guess if you hadn't fought to have the implants removed, you wouldn't be alive today."

She replied, "I don't know how much time I have left. They did some radiation treatments last May and June to help the bones and reduce the pain I was experiencing. That was okay and actually I felt pretty good until they followed that with my first and only round of chemotherapy."

"When did you have chemotherapy, Kim?" I asked.

"I had my only round of chemotherapy this past August. My white cell count went so low I was quarantined in the hospital. When John was allowed in to visit, which was only a few minutes at a time, he had to wear a gown, gloves, and a mask. I couldn't handle it. They had already told me I was going to die and I sure as hell wasn't going to die like that – alone, isolated, and in a cold sterile hospital. I refused any other chemotherapy treatments. Now, I get shots and take Oxycontin for the pain. That's it.

"I have good days and bad days. I am just thankful to have a few more days with John, and time to say good-bye to important people in my life. That is why I am so glad I found you. You know, last October I was supposed to start a job at the Treatment Center here in Page. I was going to be the head therapist."

The chill took my voice hostage. I did not know what to say. I knew she was telling the truth. I knew that stage four breast cancer meant little hope for survival. The words "I'm sorry" fell out of my mouth like golf balls clanging in a metal bucket.

"Will you come to Page and visit me? We have a beautiful home and I would love for you to come," Kim said with a bounce in her voice.

I wanted to scream, "No, I can't. I can't bear to watch you die. I am a coward. I don't want to see the ugliness of death."

But instead, I said, "Kim, we have a lot of catching up to do. You are married and I want to hear about that, and I am in a committed female relationship."

She said, "That's great; bring her. I would love to meet anyone with whom you are in love."

We talked further about her relationship and marriage to John, and I caught her up on the events in my life. I felt so sad, especially once I began to put the dates together. She and John were newlyweds. They had been married on October 15, 1999. It wasn't even six months after their marriage that she was officially diagnosed. But during the six months between her wedding and her diagnosis she was not feeling well, was tired all of time, and was in pain. I felt enraged that breast cancer could come and take Kim's life right out from under her nose, without even giving her the opportunity to fight.

As I got ready to hang up, I said, "Kim, I will come one day. I am not sure when. But until I do I would love to talk with you on the phone often, if you are up to it."

"I would love that." she said.

Over the next months, we had some very interesting phone calls. Kim always found humor in one thing or the other. She would talk about keeping in touch with me after her death, so that I could let her know when they found a cure. She told me, "They will find a cure one day. They have to. You will have to tell me all about it."

We would joke and laugh and talk about Page and Phoenix and other nonsense as we kept connected. As I got more distance from my own terror, I began to feel like I could make a visit to see Kim. I had put the visit off because I just wasn't ready to be that close to death from a disease that I also carried in my own body. Christmas came and went, and then in the spring Kim began to get worse. I made up my mind that we would go and we set a date right around Easter. The week before our visit, Kim's husband, John called and said that if I wanted to see her while she was still coherent, I had better come now.

I changed my office schedule, and Pam drove me to Page early the next morning. It was a long drive for a day trip. I had never been to Lake Powell before, but Pam used to have a boat at the lake so she was quite familiar with the long ride.

Pam dropped me off at Kim's house a bit after 11:00 a.m. Kim and her husband were expecting me. Kim was sitting up on the couch. Her hands, feet, and head shook from all of the medication she was on. Her gorgeous long hair was gone. It had been replaced with very curly hair. We talked.

I had never met John before. I noticed how attentive and gentle he was toward her. We talked about cancer: her journey with it, and mine. We talked about the inept medical field and how inadequate she felt her treatment had been. Even though I didn't ask, I wanted to know if anyone had discussed stem cell transplant with her. It didn't even seem like anyone had offered it to her or made the suggestion. Sometimes it is just too late to attempt any type of treatment.

Kim told John that she had to go to the bathroom. John helped her up with the walker. He wanted her to go to the closest one. She wanted to go all the way down the hall. I thought at first it was just her desire to prove to herself that she could make it a few more feet. In retrospect, I think she wanted to protect me from the sounds. Before John got her to the bathroom, she threw up, retching from deep inside. I just went away to that space far inside of me. The sound, the look, the smell of death, permeated every molecule of air in the house. I was frightened by the devastation but I certainly could not show it.

"Oh, God, please not me," I heard myself silently pleading. "Oh, God, please be merciful. Stop her suffering. There is just no point in this type of pain." I begged for her.

John took Kim back to her bedroom when she was done. He cleaned up the vomit and told me that she wanted to see me to say good-bye. He made a point of telling me not to stay too long because she was exhausted and had handled about all she could that day.

I went in and knelt on the floor beside her. I had brought her a rock from my special rock collection for her to hold. When I gave it to her, I told her, "Kim, this is a symbol to remind you that someone else out here in this world cares and prays for you as you make this transition to the next place."

I reminded her about a phone conversation that we had in December. During that call she told me that I would live to see a cure for cancer and when I did, I needed to come tell her all about it. During that conversation, I had asked her, "How will I recognize you when you visit me after your death?"

She reminded me of a class in which I talked about my brother. She told me she liked birds and that she would be the first bird I saw as soon as I finished a phone call with my brother. I smiled. I reminded her that day in the bedroom that I would be looking for her after those phone calls.

Now, it has been years since her death. Since that time, Kim and I have renegotiated our contract. I don't speak with my brother nearly as often as I would like, yet I find myself checking in with Kim quite often. It is amazing how aware I have become of various birds and bird behavior. I see all sorts of birds here in Arizona. I often joke with Kim when I catch a bird doing unusual things. I once watched a dove trying desperately to build a nest in an impossible place at our house. I asked Kim to please help this new momma bird. I was concerned that if she built the nest in the rain gutter the eggs would fry before hatching because of the intense Phoenix sun. So I appealed to Kim and asked her to please help this bird build a safe nest.

As I finish this book I miss Kim more than usual. I think it is time to go for a walk, talk to a bird, and check in with her. I need to see if she likes what I have written about her. I suspect her message would be something like, "Enjoy the moment; it might be your last."

CHAPTER 32

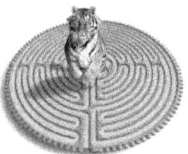

OTHER FACES ALONG MY PATH

Remembering Kim's story caused me to pause and take notice of other women with breast cancer who have crossed my path. I found it amazing that prior to my diagnosis in 1999 I knew personally only three women with the diagnosis. Two of those women were clients.

One client, Janet, had been finished with her treatment for a few years before she came to see me for psychotherapy. However, it was through Janet's story that I learned about the relationship between Tamoxifen and uterine cancer. Janet was one of those unlucky three percent of Tamoxifen users who ended up with uterine cancer. Of course, at the time of her uterine cancer, the medical field was still clueless about the relationship between Tamoxifen and uterine cancer.

It is stories like Janet's that make me aware how misleading statistical data can be. Janet's medical team didn't admit – or perhaps didn't know – that her uterine cancer was more likely than not caused by Tamoxifen. Thus, Janet's uterine cancer did not provide the medical community with statistical data because she was not part of a clinical trial. As a result of Janet's story, and the stories of hundreds of other women who were also not part of clinical trials but who developed uterine cancer while on Tamoxifen, it is realized that the real percentages are much higher than three percent.

The other client, Ann, was working with me on her family of origin material when, right in the middle of her psychotherapy, she was diagnosed with breast cancer. Ann was a vivacious, funny, and delightful woman to work with. She was serious about healing her past. She was devastated at the diagnosis. I was upset about it, too. That old script – that people who get cancer die of cancer – was not completely diminished for me with Virginia's success story. But, at least I was able to take solace from Virginia's success and share the work from **Getting Well Again** with Ann.

We blended the breast cancer healing work and Ann's family of origin work and continued to work together throughout her breast cancer treatment.

Ann's sense of humor came to the foreground concerning her baldness. I never knew what to expect when I opened the door to invite Ann into her appointment. Her hats were very entertaining, unique and expressive of her personality. When I ran my first Susan G. Komen race in 1992, it was for Ann. Ann is still alive and well today.

The third woman, Carol, was a minister at an East Coast church. We met in 1993 in Wales where we both were attending a workshop on contemplative spirituality and community building. Carol was my roommate at the conference. Carol and I remained friends and kept in contact after Wales. In 1995, we went on a week's pilgrimage together to Taos, New Mexico. We shared many of the same beliefs and enjoyed each other's conversation and spiritual discussion.

In 1997, Carol called to let me know she had been diagnosed with breast cancer and was scheduled for a mastectomy.

Carol was already familiar with visualization work and she used stars to assist her in her healing imagery. She sent stars throughout her whole body, letting them build up the white blood cells, and infiltrate and attach the mutant cancer cells. During Carol's treatment, I offered up healing prayers, and sent her star symbols to encourage her in her work.

Since my diagnosis in 1999, I have been inundated with friends and family who have been diagnosed. Denise, Pam's sister-in-law, was diagnosed in April of 2000. She had her biopsy and got her diagnosis on the same day I had my hysterectomy. Closely connected with me have been Denise, Shirley, Lynn, Kim, Veronica, Jude, Teri, Cindy, and Carol. Lynn, Kim, and Jude are gone. Lynn was a former student diagnosed at about the same time as I was. She had stage four breast cancer. Kim and Jude both had inflammatory breast cancer.

Currently, I have other clients and dear friends who have been diagnosed with various stages of breast cancer or other forms of horrific cancer. Their stories are relevant and still in the making. During each psychotherapy session, I observe something new about myself. I see my client's courage amidst their fear. I hear their terror beneath their hope. I learn that I too am courageous and have been able to make meaning out of this journey for myself. We all belong to an infantry of soldiers that must keep watch over our own bodies. Each story becomes a nugget of hope and I carry that hope with me throughout the day.

In 1999, the statistics on breast cancer claimed that three of eight people who get breast cancer die from it. Those statistics seem to be accurate in my circle of acquaintances. Three of the original eight women who I knew are gone. Breast cancer as portrayed in the Susan G. Komen races affects everyone in some way. It is epidemic. If you have never attended a Susan G. Komen Race for the Cure, treat yourself this year by attending one in your area. If you have not experienced the race, you truly do not know what you are missing. You can participate by walking, running, volunteering or by being the loudest cheerleader from the hundreds of people on the sidelines. I can almost promise that you will encounter an experience that will enrich your life and change it in subtle or even dramatic ways.

Somewhere along this breast cancer journey I read a statement that made me smile. Some doctor made a statement, "Women with breast cancer have melancholy personalities." The statement certainly struck me as an overgeneralization and I was not sure where he was gathering his facts. But, when you attend a Susan G. Komen race, you see an ocean of pink-shirt survivors fighting, singing, running, and dancing for their lives. There is nothing melancholy about that group.

CHAPTER 33

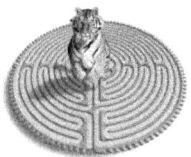

FINISHING UNFINISHED BUSINESS

I wish that my being a psychologist fixed all of my personality quirks before granting me a degree, sort of like the game Monopoly where you can draw a "get out of jail" free card. But it doesn't. I have my share of baggage, deficiencies, and rough edges. Adding those endearing qualities to personal needs, ideals, and goals can lead to troubled waters.

Prior to the diagnosis of breast cancer, my life had been tremendously rewarding. I believe I had accomplished many things for a Southern mill town girl. My extensive travels took me to many countries, allowing me to reside in places like Australia, New Zealand, and Western Samoa. I also lived for several years in Hawaii, both on the Big Island of Hawaii and on Oahu. Those travels encompassed my first few years after graduating from high school when I served with the religious organization Youth With A Mission.

Following my work with Youth With A Mission, I spent fourteen years in church-related work on Whidbey Island in Washington State. It was there that I began my academic education and my practice in psychology. However, after fourteen years on a small, twenty-one mile island I became antsy to move. In 1987 an opportunity to relocate to Phoenix, Arizona presented itself to me. Just like all of my prior moves, my heart awakened and I knew that Phoenix would be the next chapter in my life. I came here to be part of a dynamic ministry, Iverna Tompkins' Ministries. At that time, Iverna Tompkins' Ministries provided intensive workshops, trainings, and spiritual rehabilitation for clergy and their families. I spent two years working with clergy from across the country and assisting them in building healthy ministerial relationships. Iverna was a delight to work with and I felt deeply honored and blessed to be part of her team and vision for God's people, but I found myself lonely for my Episcopal community.

One of the first professional relationships that I developed here was with an Episcopal priest. I met Matthew at an AIDS conference and we immediately connected. We made arrangements to have lunch and the lunch ended up in a job opportunity for me. I worked with Matthew designing and implementing a training program for lay Eucharistic ministers in the Episcopal Diocese of Arizona. That collegial relationship grew into a friendship that was very significant for me, and I considered Matthew a best friend, spiritual mentor, and a great colleague. The Eucharist is one of the most important parts of my spiritual life. It is a cornerstone of the beliefs of the Episcopal people. For several years I worked side by side with Matthew providing training for lay Eucharistic ministers. Once the participants completed their training, these "non-ordained" lay people then were equipped to take the Eucharist to the sick and shut-in within their different parishes.

Within two years of Matthew's and my friendship, two other priests moved to town. One became the priest of the parish church I attended and his wife filled multiple jobs within the diocese. We lived near each other, and soon became good friends. Jeff and Susan trusted me and shared much of their pain from their past parish experience with me. For a couple of years, everything went along just fine. I had my own little safe haven within our Episcopal community. Then leadership in the church changed when a new bishop moved to town. As time went on, things fell apart between the new bishop and Matthew. And as in most situations such as this one, things between people became nasty. My loyalty pulled and pushed me, tossing and turning my soul, tearing holes of resentment, anger, unrest, judgment, and confusion.

I remember the phone call. "Robin, this is Matthew."

"Hey, what's up?" I asked.

The specific details of the conversation that followed are not my story to tell. But my inner feelings became a tidal wave of emotional chaos. I allowed myself to be swept away with its pain. My loyalty to Matthew rose up. I was off with my own conclusions and judgments.

As a result, I cut off my friendship with Susan. I wasn't even very civil around her. I was like an ice queen. I turned my focus to other things when I had to communicate with her. I was professional and business-like, but never bothered with even the most simple pleasantries of "Hi, how are you?" I looked through her instead of at her. I talked at her instead of to her. Thankfully, I had the wherewithal to keep my mouth shut and not triangulate mutual friends into the private battle I was having with Susan. But I grew bitter toward her and that bitterness was fed each time I saw her.

I had continued to do some teaching in the diocese even after Matthew left. I did not pursue those teaching opportunities and at times felt hypocritical teaching there with so much resentment. Thankfully the bitterness never superseded my sanity and I refused to stop doing what I loved just because of my issues with Susan.

Then when Dr. West said, "Ms. Dilley, I am sorry you have breast cancer," amazingly enough the bell in the boxing match rang, and I knew clearly I was in need of forgiveness. God obviously knew that, too.

In October of 1999, I was scheduled to teach a Friday night and all day Saturday workshop for the new deacons. I knew Susan would be around as she always was when I taught. So I called Susan and told her I would like some private time to speak with her. "I need to ask you to forgive me and I want to do that in person."

I did not have to explain myself. My cold, aloof actions were not misunderstood by her. She knew I blamed her for Matthew's leaving without me having to tell her. That Saturday during lunch I accompanied her to the privacy of her office. There I said, "Susan, it is no secret between us that I have blamed you for Matthew's departure. I do not need to nor want to go into any of that story. What I do need and want is your forgiveness. I have been cold, curt, and at times nasty with you. I ask you to forgive me. I picked up a battle that was not mine to fight. It was clearly none of my business. I have judged you harshly and resented you. Please forgive me."

Through her gentle smile and soft eyes we saw each other again, no longer looking past or through each other but into each other's soul. She said, "Robin, I forgave you a long time ago and it is very meaningful to me that you can walk back into my life. I have missed our friendship and want it back again."

I, of course, was crying. We prayed together. I went back to teach the afternoon session much lighter than I had been for years. Susan's friendship has grown steadily since that October day in 1999 and I am thankful that I finished my unfinished business and am alive to tell the story.

Hurt – emotional hurt – is one of the most misunderstood entities in our culture. Unfortunately, we passively assume that people who build judgments and resentments, host angers and jealousies, and are hostile are bad people. The reality is that harsh behaviors in any person always have hurt behind them. Anger and resentment are debilitating coping devices that make the problem worse instead of better. As humans, we all struggle with these powerful and debilitating emotions.

When I was feeling anger and resentment towards Susan, I was deeply uncomfortable with such strong negative emotions and feelings about a fellow human being, a former friend. But I was protected. No one was going to get into my armor and touch me in such a way that I would hurt again. I was not going to lose another friendship because of someone else. I was not going to look at reason or rationale, or accept any explanation. I was in my four-year-old ego state that was screaming, "You hurt my buddy, and I hate you."

The armor of my four-year-old was strong, secure, and safe. I stayed there, hiding behind it like a child in a tree house refusing to come down regardless of how cold or hungry I became. Thankfully, because of my understanding of psychological dynamics, I understood in hindsight that losses of significant people in my life take me right back to that young four- or five-year-old ego state when Matt moved away and I was left with an angry, hateful, skinny white woman as my caretaker.

My loyalty surrounding Matthew became damaging from that early childhood wound of loss. My castle became fortified with a demanding four-year-old who screamed, "You can't make me. I don't like you." My old coping and adapting strategies of the child/me had taken over. I was not operating from my adult ego state, but from that hurt inner child state.

From a psychological perspective, that wounded ego state needed to be healed, provided for, listened to, and made to feel safe in her loss. Once that happened, the four-year-old loved (as four-year-olds do) to make new friends, see new things, and fix broken hearts.

When I asked for forgiveness, I knew I was holding my adult self accountable for giving into the actions of my four-year-old. I knew that my four-year-old needed my understanding and empathy for the mess I allowed her to make out of my friendship with Susan. I knew and understood that the process of forgiveness in this situation was about taking responsibility for my actions and beliefs.

It is a much clearer picture, when asking for forgiveness, not to explain your actions, not to excuse them in any way, but to say forthrightly and directly, "I hurt you. I was cold, curt, and mean. I am sorry. Will you forgive me?"

CHAPTER 34

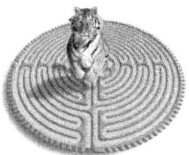

OTHER SPIRITUAL PIECES:
THE LABYRINTH

My life has always been a mixed tapestry of spirituality. Spirituality is a part of who I am and not something that I do. I deeply believe that we are spiritual beings and it is our job to attend to our spiritual garden. The spiritual garden is within each of us and we can let it grow weeds, let it dry up and die, or we can gently tend to it throughout all of the days of our lives. When we face a storm our garden can become overwhelmed with waves and wind damage and we must use our resources to repair it and re-establish it. When there is a drought we must carry water to our spiritual garden. In the next few chapters, I want to share some of the spiritual practices that I used during and after my journey with breast cancer. It was natural for me to turn to my spiritual resources during this time. The Labyrinth, the Healing Power of a Native Sweat, and a Vision Quest are three key components of my journey.

During the Nineties the spiritual significance of the labyrinth began pouring into print. It seemed that everywhere I turned someone was writing or talking about their experience of God as he or she walked the labyrinth. I began to read about this spiritual practice and discovered its ancient history. A labyrinth is not a maze. In the English language the words "labyrinth" and "maze" are often used interchangeably. A maze contains dead ends and often has many entrances. A labyrinth has one entrance and one exit. It is a path from the outside in and then from the inside out. It has a sacred sense of journey about it; perhaps the eleven-circuit labyrinth began as a spiritual practice for those who could not make the annual pilgrimage to Jerusalem. No one really knows the reason labyrinths were created but there are eleven-circuit and seven-circuit labyrinths. Seven-circuit labyrinths date back four to five thousand years and are seen in Hopi, Cretan, and Celtic spiritual practices. The most famous eleven-circuit labyrinth is in Chartres Cathedral in Chartres, France, and dates back to the twelfth century. The number of circuits simply means the number of times the pilgrim passes the center of the labyrinth during his or her walk.

My interest in the labyrinth grew. I responded to that interest by making a special pilgrimage to San Francisco to walk the labyrinth at Grace Cathedral. There, I, too, experienced a peaceful sense of purpose. I felt a sense of holiness about the journey in and out and around the path that brings us into the center of God, and back out to the world again. Grace Cathedral has an indoor and an outdoor eleven-circuit labyrinth. The indoor one provides the pilgrim with quite an intense experience because sacred music is playing during the labyrinth walk. It was easy for me as I walked it to become lost in the music, feeling as if I was transcending consciousness. The outdoor labyrinth overlooked the busy San Francisco streets. Walking it created a sense of purpose, with a special connection to the world. The two labyrinths provided me with an experience and a picture of God inside of me and outside of me at the same time.

When I left San Francisco, I wanted desperately to have a local labyrinth. I felt a strange loneliness for it. I felt connected, sort of called to it as a way of worship. There was something about this walking meditation that provided me with an experience of God that fed my hungry soul. That journey to San Francisco was in 1997.

In 1998 our Episcopal Cathedral, Trinity, was under reconstruction. Trinity is a local historical landmark for Phoenix as well as the headquarters for the Episcopal bishop and church administration. The Dean of the cathedral at the time, Rev. Rebecca McClain, was in charge of the reconstruction. Lo and behold, she was having a beautiful eleven-circuit labyrinth built in the center of the courtyard. I felt like God had answered my prayers. I was ecstatic about the plans. I couldn't wait for it to be finished. Trinity finished the labyrinth in December 2000. One of my New Year's resolutions of 2001 was to walk the labyrinth once a week for the entire year.

I walked it every Wednesday. If I was out of town for some reason, I made arrangements to walk it at some other time. The experience of that commitment created a sacred space inside of me and I developed a personal relationship with this sacred art form that allowed me to be touched and touch God in unique ways. I was very aware during my labyrinth walks of the gift of life. It seemed that each week my gratitude for my life and my recovery became deeper. I was aware on these walks with God that my life was meaningful and that I needed to be awake to all God had in store for me. During this time my gratitude for being alive grew.

I definitely have an attention problem that becomes a bother in times of prayer, but the motion of walking, following a path, and making a pilgrimage to the center where all is well and perfect is a powerful and unifying experience. I used this time with God to refocus my life, to pull close to the spiritual world, recommitting to a life of meaningful experience with God. I not only re-dedicated my life to one of service and ministry but also used the time to refocus on the art of prayer and watched as my prayer life transformed from a dead stick in the ground to a beautiful lush green plant.

The story of the dead stick is significant because when I was a student of spiritual direction during my master's program, I had a director who told me to plant a stick in the ground and to water and care for it as if it were alive. Of course, I thought this was a silly exercise, but part of being a student of spiritual direction is learning to follow direction. I learned so much from this exercise that it still empowers my conscious-ness in my psychotherapy practice. For example, many times I think to myself, we are not getting anywhere in therapy. Nothing is ever going to change in this person's life; it is just the same old thing. In my discouragement it would be easy to give up, but I remember the exercise of watering the stick. This mutually powerful and silly exercise taught me to stay with a project even though it seems fruitless.

The stick did not change, but I did. I learned just how much water the earth was able to absorb in order for the stick not to get too wet and rot. I also had to learn just how much water was sufficient to keep the ground closed around the stick in order that it remained erect. I practiced caring for it daily while acknowledging that I got nothing back in return. I had to live through my own embarrassment about the craziness of watering a stick, thinking horribly judgmental thoughts at times. Sometimes, those judgmental thoughts were directed at me and my stupidity for participating in such a ridiculous exercise and at other times those criticisms were directed at my spiritual director.

In my head, I accused her of being mean and manipulative. Walking the labyrinth on a weekly basis sometimes was like watering the stick. Sometimes I felt silly, as if I were going nowhere. At other times, it was a soul-ripping experience that shook me to my core. I was able to unravel complexities in my life during that time. I was able to pick up pieces of my life that I had laid aside, such as my writing. I was able to focus again on the alpha and omega of God. At the same time that I started my relationship with the labyrinth, I also started a professional relationship with a teacher and healer.

CHAPTER 35

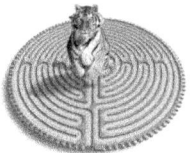

MY WORK WITH DR. H

My interest in Native American and shamanic practices continually tugged at my heart. I kept my eyes and ears open for more opportunities, but it wasn't until 1996 when I took a three- month sabbatical to work on a novel (that still lays in the bottom drawer of my filing cabinet) that I came across the name, "Dr. Carl Hammerschlag." He had a project called Turtle Island. I drafted him a letter. I am not sure I ever sent it. I wanted desperately to discover all of the magic inside of me and learn what I could about shamanism. As I said in the chapter about the Mercury Fantasy Camp and playing HORSE with Jennifer Gillom, breast cancer gave me the courage to do things that I would not ordinarily do.

Even though I was two years post active treatment for my breast cancer, I was still actively seeking all avenues of healing. Therefore I felt it necessary to act on the long ignored urge to do some personal work with Dr. Hammerschlag. In January of 2001, I called Dr. Hammerschlag and made an appointment to see him for individual psychotherapy. Sitting with him was like entering a magical place where the ordinary becomes extraordinary, where the curtain between the natural and the supernatural split, allowing me to see the ordinarily invisible, hear the unexpected, and practice ritual that created meaning in my life.

Seeing "Dr. H", as I fondly call him, enhanced my practice of spirituality and gave me permission to live my life in wild abandonment. I saw him during the time I was also walking the labyrinth weekly. It is a lonely world out here in this spiritual plane, and having someone help facilitate the journey made it easier, more satisfying, and less solitary. Through Dr. H's encouragement and his connections to his many Native American relatives, I had an opportunity to go to a healing sweat.

Sweat lodges are a traditional healing practice in most Native American tribes. Willow branches or other flexible wood is used to build a round dome-like structure that is then covered with blankets. The door to the sweat opens to the east, which is the direction God dwells in most cultures. In the center of the sweat is a two-foot-deep hole. Then hot stones, which are referred to as our *ancestors*, are placed ritually in that hole. The ceremony consists of four rounds. At the beginning of each round, new stones, hot with fire from the fire pit, are brought to the center of the sweat. An altar which holds sage, cedar, and other sacred objects of the clan or tribe holding the sweat rests between the fire pit and the door to the sweat. The purpose of a sweat is for purification and healing. Any time you are invited to participate in a sweat you are being treated as family, part of the tribe. It is a sacred honor. A medicine man or woman should facilitate any sweat that you attend.

I do not feel that just telling you about the experience of the sweat is sufficient. As I struggled with this chapter trying to keep a sense of aliveness to it I made the decision to share some of the prose I wrote the day after my sweat lodge experience. These words portray as adequately as possible my experience. Please do not try to understand them, but try to join me in allowing yourself to experience the words.

Sacred Ground

I enter.
I notice the desert dust, the native trees, and the indigenous shrubs.
I wait.
I imagine what today will bring.

They appear, as magic dropped from heaven's cloud. No one, and all of a

sudden,   everyone.
They speak their names and their tribe.
I feel embarrassed. I have no tribe.

She comes toward me in her native attire full of symbolic life,
Medicine Woman, the answer to a very old and tired prayer.
Time parts and we enter a Holy Place. Dialogue occurs.
Surreal, the earth I am standing on shifts, I am here and there, at the same
time.

I watch as another younger Medicine Woman places carefully and ceremoni-
ously sacred items, on the flesh of Mother Earth around the Turtle's head. I do
not know…I do not need to know in order for me to respect and honor. I now
know why none of this is written in books for white people. I now know this
Holy Place by touch and by taste.

She speaks, I listen.

I stand, and the Tender of the Fire ushers cedar blessings to dance around my
body.
I enter, clockwise and sit by Medicine Woman as she directs. Other women
enter. The Keeper of the Fire brings in the ancestors, the stones, nine of them,
they call the stones the Ancient Ones. Cedar blesses each of them.

I am anxious, tight, but wanting, yearning, in need of a sacrament for heal-
ing.
She talks with me carefully, almost in a cadence, a rhythm of her own. She
has been up all night to a special meeting. I suspect she is still in trance. She
then asks that I share my name and my story.

I share my first name only, unaware that she needs my surname. I give a
skeleton sketch of my story and why I am here today.

Next, Medicine is explained and Tobacco is passed. She prays. I pray. To-

bacco blesses me. We pray. We pray for each other. There are 11 of us – nine adults and two children.

The medicine in the water is given to the ancestors. The ancestors breathe on us with their breath. Heat begins to purify. The praying continues and then magically stops. The curtain opens. Cool air brushes against my sweat. I relax.

The curtain closes again. It opens and shuts three more times. I know there will be four rounds. Each time something more and uncommon happens. This time different medicine is passed. It is blessed by the Keeper of the Fire. She takes two spoonfuls, places it in the palm of her hand and eats it. Just like communion. I can do this. Water from the teepee is passed. We wash the medicine down with the teepee water. Just like the holy Eucharist, the Body and Blood of Christ. The Medicine that is being passed is in a jar. It appears to be green in color and very granular. Each woman prays before she eats it. I watch. I have heard of this medicine. I now know something unusual and sacred is happening. They are sharing what I understand to be their most Holy Medicine, their sacrament, with me of No Tribe. I feel deeply honored. The Medicine comes to me, this Medicine that the Keeper of the Fire has passed to all. I take two spoonfuls. I look at it. I pray too, inside and quietly. I ask the Medicine to be gentle with me and treat me kindly. I remind the Medicine I have no tribe and am in need of healing. I ask the Medicine to bring me what I need. I take the Medicine. It is dense, grainy, expands in my mouth. I have some around my lips. Thank God for my teachings. I know it is Sacred. I know I must get the Medicine from around my lips into my mouth. I know all Medicine must be licked from my hand as well. I know this intrinsically and had trained laity on how to take the Sacrament to those homebound and in hospitals. I know the Blood of Christ must be given back to the earth and not poured down a drain. I know the blessed Body of Christ must be fully consumed. I understand Sacrament and always intrinsically have. It is my bloodline, from some ancient one.

I pass the jar on. I attend to getting the entire Sacrament in my mouth. The teepee water is passed. I do not know what or how it was used in ritual the night before, but I know it is blessed. I allow the teepee water to swirl in mouth, catching the dancing granules and carry it to the rest of my body. Everyone has partaken. The children left to play at the end of the first round. I know if they had been there they, too, would have partaken. Everyone has tasted of the Sacrament. The curtain closes. The Medicine Woman begins to pour water on the ancient ones. Now there are 18 stones in the center. The Keeper of the Fire is in charge of praying during this round. She begins to pray and the other, younger Medicine Woman plays the drum. It becomes very loud, very hot. Very surreal. Where am I and in what time zone? It is dark. Magically the praying stops and the curtain again opens. Cool air comes and melts against my sweaty body.

I know this is no ordinary day and not just another Sweat.

The Medicine woman turns to me. She tells me the story of her traveling to the desert of the Southwest. She tells me the miracle of her daughter's birth. Her daughter now 19 is lying with her head in the lap of the woman from the Cree nation. Her daughter has been ill for days with the flu. Her daughter is quietly listening as her mother tells me her birth story and of her naming. Her mother also tells me of her husband. A medicine man. She tells me how she misses him. She cries. I listen. I know this is about story. I know this is about relatives and connection. I know this is about my own mother and her story of me and the story of my naming. I miss my mother intensely as Medicine Woman talks. I see images of my mother and me. I am reminded of the sacredness between us and between a Mother and Daughter. And too I am reminded of the pain of disconnection. The disconnection that leaves its scar and allows me to grieve my losses. I, too, cry. I cry tears for my mother.

The Keeper of the Fire is bringing in nine more stones as the Medicine Woman tells her story. The Cedar blesses the ancient ones. The one from the Navaho nation is asked to pray during this round. She accepts the praying stick. It has been here the whole time. I just now notice it. The Navaho tells us she will pray in her native tongue. She begins. The drumming begins. It gets loud, dark, and hotter. Then I see her. There she is. I know her. I am aware. I cry. I dialogue with her. She speaks; I listen.

Then the chanting stops. The drum continues for a bit. The curtain opens. The cool air comes in and nourishes my hot and sweaty body. I am asked how I am doing. Another story is told while nine more rocks are brought in. The prayer stick is handed back to the Medicine Woman. The curtain closes and the prayers begin. As she pours the water on the now 36 ancestors, the heat rises fast. This time it is burning. My lips, my knuckles, my knees next to the stones. Everything burns....I know this is the fire of purification. I breathe its heat into my lungs. I pray for purification, forgiveness, wisdom, and healing. I pray in my prayer language, the one I received earlier in my youth; it is an ancient spiritual language, from some other place. I don't care anymore. All inhibitions have been burned off. My body feels as if it is in a spasm from the hotness of the fire. The burning goes deeper. The pain inten-sifies. I feel like I am enveloped in the flame. I feel as if I am in the middle of the fire. It is burning from me those trappings that need to go. I pray to be purified. To be touched by the Holy One. I imagine going into the fire. There are those arms. They hold me. I am okay. I listen now. I hear the prayers, the drum. It stops. The curtain opens for the fourth and final time. I exit into the coolness. The sun shines gently. A soft breeze wipes my sweat. I look and my legs are very red. I know this heat. I am aware.

I lie on Mother Earth.   I notice my relatives and all living things around me have changed. The dust of the desert, Creator God's blanket. The native trees are watching over us. The indigenous plants offer their life so that we may live in wholeness.

I have been touched by Creator Mother-Father God today. The rocks, the trees, the shrubs and the dust connect my soul to these ancient wise ones. I have entered a dif-ferent space, a different time, but yet have always been here. I now see. Thank you Creator Mother – Father God. Thank you, Medicine Woman and my sisters.

Afterwards, we eat together, dishes brought and made. It is one daughter's birthday. Cake and ice cream are shared. The surreal feeling stays, stuck to me like a warm wet coat. I smile. I talk to my new sisters. I play with the children. Life wants to appear normal again. It never will. I wonder about cake and ice cream. I wonder if there is a history to this tradition or if we just do it. White pale faced Anglos, descendants of the Celtic nation. Lost history. In need of wholeness.

I drive home. I am still entranced. I carry with me the one who came. I talk with her. She talks with me. I know her. She arrived in 1996. I have had only brief dialogues with her. She has sent others. Teachers. The Favored One. Firewoman, The Muse. She has sent them all. I have not done well in honoring them. I become entrapped in the casings of daily life.

Breast Cancer came. I embraced it as a teacher. I worked with it with the Favored One and my totem Tiger. Half of my breast is gone, replaced by a scar. The scar, like those of my youth is a reminder of my history, the place from which I come. Our scars are reminders of how strong we really are and how mysterious Mother-Father God is. How out of all of the past stories, the Southern history, the embers of healing wait patiently for us to tend to them. I reflect on their culture and then my own. Meaning – deep meaning – comes from doing the journey.

On the drive home, I notice nothing outside of my internal process. The process deep, entranced, Holy. More writing will flow. My muse has not forsaken me.

I exit the new roundabout. The sky is pink; creamy flashes of thick clouds melt into the dusk. I am grateful.

I arrive home. Life on the outside appears to be the same. On the inside, it is different.

This day and its essence will teach me for many moons to come.

This day will stand out in my life, always. The essence of this day will quicken my soul every day of my days to come. I am different. Life is different.

That sweat's essence still feeds me today. I recall, remember, and recount the exchange and use its energy to move me forward in my life. My work with Dr. H is a gift I give which allows me to stay focused, balanced and on my journey. I desire to stay awake to the magic, the mystery of life.

CHAPTER 36

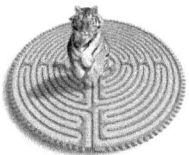

OTHER POWERFUL CEREMONIES OF LIFE

The link between the spiritual, the mystical, the magical, and the energy that makes the ordinary extraordinary has called to me from my earliest memories. I have always had an interest in Native American stories, rituals, and ceremonies. Perhaps that interest grew from the simplest of childhood rituals. My mother, whose middle name was Noka (said to be an Indian name), used to entertain my cousin, Michael, and me with Indian stories. My mother would make a circle, build a small fire in the middle of it, then call us to come and sit around the fire. There she told us stories, none of which I remember. However, I do recall vividly the experience of sitting on the grass, the coolness of the evening, the fire in the circle, and the delight in my mother's voice as she wove the words, mesmerizing us into entering some make-believe world of the unknown.

When I moved to Washington State, I discovered Carlos Castaneda's books as well as other books on shamanism and Native American spirituality. Then when I arrived in the Valley of the Sun, I felt like I had been dropped from the spirit of the Northwest Indian to the spiritual energy of the grand Southwest Indians – the Hopi, Pima, Yavapai, Navaho, Apache, and the Yaqui. It seemed that everywhere I turned I was drawn to their stories and ceremonies.

For instance, in 1992 I was invited to attend an Apache ceremony for a young girl becoming a woman – "na'ii'ees" as it is called in its native language. This "changing woman" ceremony was another life-changing event for me. The Apache Sunrise Ceremony is an arduous communal ceremony where the young Apache girl upon her first menses participates in a four-day ritual of song, prayers, dance, and running in four directions. The North, East, South, and West are sacred points on the Native American medicine wheel and those directions are honored during various Native ceremonies. The young woman goes without food and is flocked on her right and her left by her godmother and a medicine man. Another girl child, an older sister or cousin, also dances beside her, holding a cup of water with a straw. The young assistant gives the water to the changing woman throughout the hours of dance, and offers encouragement and support throughout the long and intricate rituals. The changing woman never holds nor touches the cup. She is only allowed to touch the straw to her lips.

After dancing for three days, the ceremony ends as the young woman runs in the sacred four directions offering prayers and enacting the four phases of life – childhood, youth, adulthood, and the age of the crone, the old wise one. Then the celebration of food and gifts begins.

The history of this ceremony and the one for the Navaho women, "kinaalda," was severely damaged when the U.S. government banned all Native American spiritual practices in the 1900s. By making the ceremony an illegal act, the government actively participated in the demise of a deeply spiritual nation, causing shame, abandonment, fear, and a lack of personal pride to settle in like a deep sleep over a people who were in tune with changing seasons and changing phases of life. It wasn't until 1978 when the American Indian Religious Freedom Act was passed that the changing woman ceremony and many others were re-established.

Seventy-eight years of history had been lost by that time and a ritual that brought so much to its people had to be rebirthed, and the people of the tribe re-educated about the power and significance of such a ritual. How the Native culture survived such abuse is a miracle in and of itself and a testimony to the endurance of the human spirit. As a breast cancer survivor I relate to that endurance. The U.S. government, like Hitler, tried to wipe out an entire nation of people. But they survived. Cancer's mission is to wipe out our body's ability to resist, fight, and recover. But when we do overcome, a powerful story of strength is born.

As I stood in the unrelenting hot sun watching this young Apache girl dance, dressed in her native apparel of buckskin, feathers, and symbolic beads and jewelry, I marveled at the young girl's fortitude and courage. I couldn't help wondering how life might be different for all the children of America if ceremonies such as these were provided to teach them endurance, strength, and courage.

This rite of passage develops a fortified sanctity that enriches the life of the changing woman by the act of re-enacting the creation myth and personifying White Painted Woman. White Painted Woman is the female deity who gave birth to the Son of Water and another son, Killer of Enemies. From the re-enactment of this story, the Apache girl learns to overcome her own weaknesses and dark forces, and gain strength and knowledge of her own spiritual power to bless others and practice goodness. The exhilaration of completing such a difficult task leaves the child behind and opens the door to the many manifestations of womanhood, such as creator, mother, healer, and hard worker. The after effects of this ceremony made me yearn for more understanding, participation, and connection with those who knew, loved and served the same God as I did, but in so many different ways.

CHAPTER 37

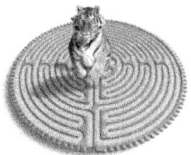

A SUBURBAN WOMAN'S MODIFIED VISION QUEST

About a year after my sweat lodge experience, I felt a strong need to get away for a few days and try to capture my story. I often go to solitary places when I am seeking direction in my life and try to figure out the answers to the questions on my heart. At this time, I was three years out from my treatment and knew I would be on Tamoxifen and have regular blood draws over the next two years. I sensed within me that it was time to capture and articulate my breast cancer journey. I wanted to find a way to intersperse this experience in my life, sort of like making sure this part of my life's tapestry had a space inside of me.   I guess I was searching for some way to make meaning out of what happened to me. I decided that it would be good for me to try to replicate a Native American tradition called a Vision Quest.

It is common in native cultures for individuals to go on a "Vision Quest." It is one of the oldest traditions used by Native people to seek direction in their life. The Native seeker usually experiences the Vision Quest under the direction of a medicine man or woman. The seeker goes "to the mountain" and spends three to four days in a blessed circle, seeking personal direction to a question or guidance for an important decision he/she needs to make. The seeker usually fasts from food and some seekers fast from water. It often reminds me of Jesus' forty days in the wilderness where he neither ate food nor drank water. Often during this arduous task the seeker becomes very sick or terrorized and afraid of dying. It is during this terror that the seeker is confronted with his or her demons inside of him/herself. Often, the seeker will have nighttime dreams or daytime visions.

In addition, animals will come to the seeker. The seeker then has to discern what messages the animal is bringing to him or her. The seeker stays in one place for at least three nights and then finds his/her way back to his/her people. The seeker holds the vision close to his/her chest. With daily gratitude, the seeker asks for wisdom to carry out the vision that was granted during the Vision Quest.

In this type of traditional Vision Quest, the seeker can be proud of him or herself for finishing such a grueling and often terrifying ritual. The seeker actually has more ego strength or personal power because of the "growing up" that happens on the quest. The quest also is "concretized," which means it becomes more real because the village celebrates with the seeker when he/she returns. Native peoples have a strong sense of respect for their communities and connections to each other and Mother Earth.

I prepared for my Vision Quest by choosing a space that allowed me to have a sense of being away and remote. It didn't take me long to remember that the Biosphere project in the middle of the Catalina Mountains might be the perfect place. The Catalina Mountains are in Southern Arizona near Tucson. When I was a doctoral student I went to a symposium that was held at the Biosphere. I fell in love with the space and always remembered it as a sacred space.

Briefly, the Biosphere was a science program in the remote desert where scientists attempted to replicate life on earth inside of this dome-like structure. When the scientists lived at the Biosphere, they had very basic individual dorm rooms. After the scientists left the project, those rooms were turned into basic guest's rooms consisting of a desk, a bed, a microwave and a small fridge. There were no TV's or telephones in the rooms, no maid service, no hotel staff except the person at the front desk during business hours. After five o'clock, you were on your own. The rooms seemed hidden away in the womb of the Catalinas.

The week before my quest, I prepared myself by cleansing my body with a detox fast. I ate only brown rice, vegetables and fruit for seven days. Preparing one's spirit to receive guidance from the "Other" means setting aside your life as you normally would live it. During that week, I also organized for my quest by carefully choosing music that I thought would feed my spirit. I did not want to be easily distracted during my quest; thus I allowed myself to take only one book and a journal for writing. Even though I knew I would be writing, I did not take my laptop computer. The actual experience of writing "longhand" uses the brain differently than typing on the keyboard. I wanted to let my body return to that process.

I packed plenty of water, comfortable clothes, comfortable shoes, fresh fruit, vegetables, peanut butter and canned beans for protein. I did not plan to eat at the restaurant on the property because that would distract me from the solitude of the Quest.

I also thoughtfully selected several items to make my space sacred. I chose sage, sweet grass, a tiger candle and a drum. I also took tobacco to mindfully sprinkle around my surroundings and a special abalone shell where I could safely burn my sage and sweet grass. I took one bowl, one cup, one fork, and one spoon. I cut down to the very basics and mindfully packed each item as if to personally invite it along for my journey.

The most important item that I took was my journal. It was there that I recorded all of the events of the quest. The careful recording of the events, the animals, the thoughts, dreams, and ideas that came to me during the quest helped me work with them for months after my quest ended. Also, by maintaining an adequate record, I was able to defend myself against any doubts that came up after the quest. I find that it only takes a few days of being back in the ordinary for self-doubt to sink in. I find those thoughts, like "*Are you kidding yourself? You are not really supposed to write a book about your journey with breast cancer*" can be very self-defeating unless I return to the pages of that journal that remind me that all I did for three days and nights was to write about my journey with breast cancer.

Because this was my own rendition of a Vision Quest, I was careful to pay close attention to what the universe brought to me. The Sunday before I departed, I started my vegetable and rice fast. On that same Sunday, Pam and I walked in the desert near us. Usually we don't see snakes in the desert and consider ourselves lucky when we see a snake's path. But, on this Sunday, Pam looked down at a bush as we were walking past it. There she saw a diamondback rattlesnake nicely curled, enjoying the morning sun. She stopped me, and we visited with the snake for the longest time. I knew it was a sign to me about my quest. I felt I was to be present and watch respectfully all that would take place on my quest. A snake in Native American tradition symbolizes transmutation, shedding one's old skin and becoming something new.

The following Sunday I started out early for my three-hour drive to the Biosphere. After I exited from the freeway the last hour was quite desolate. The curvy roads, cattle guards, and the desolation of the quiet and serene desert landscape captured my focus as excitement began to build within me. I became eager to arrive. The drive was so desolate, I thought I was never going to get there, and then mysteriously and magically, I rounded the last curve and right in front of me was the astounding Biosphere structure. The Biosphere was recently voted by Time Life Books as one of the fifty must-see wonders of the world. I knew that I had entered a different reality far away from the conveniences of the American everyday lifestyle.

After checking in at the registration desk, I found my room, and unloaded my car. Then I opened the curtains to the mountains, took a deep breath, opened the door to the patio, and stepped out to those nurturing, loving Catalina Mountains as if to say, "Here I am God." I sat for quite awhile and just drank in the experience of the mountains. Then I went inside to be settled. I took off my watch and placed it in a safe place because I did not want to march to the restrictions or demands of time. I wanted to develop my own rhythms of sleeping and eating and follow the pace that would come naturally after about the first eighteen hours of being there.

I knew I wanted to pay attention to the animals that appeared, the dreams that I might have, and any random thought that wanted to pass through my head. I might then choose to dismiss most random thoughts but I did not want to miss anything that might be coming my way. As I was unpacking, I heard sounds beneath my room. The brush was rattling beneath the deck. Venturing out and looking over the banister, I discovered a herd of desert pigs. In the Southwest those pigs are called Javelinas. Under my deck there were babies, mommas, and a few very heavy, very old-looking Javelinas that had discovered a nice cool place to lie down. It was September, but September is still very hot in Arizona. Other Javelinas went completely under the deck. I could no longer see some of them but I certainly could hear them snorting and grunting below. At that moment, I knew the Universe was making my Vision Quest sacred. I was being welcomed into the sacred where I believed I could expect good things. I continued to sit on the patio, watch, and write for several hours.

As evening cast its shadowy light, I could hear water running in the distance from a small spring that ran through the property. I left my room and took a nice long walk around the area. I walked around the "lungs" of the biosphere and felt sad that the project had been abandoned. The grounds were lush green and the evening temperature was perfect. In the distance appeared three small deer. They were coming to get a drink of water. I just stood still and watched. Darkness closed in around the light of the day and it was time for me to head for my room. I continued to write in my journal, prepared a small dinner of fresh vegetables and beans, and then read until sleep overtook me.

Dawn arrived and the gentle light found its way through my curtains. I stirred, prepared myself some hot tea, and returned to my balcony.

The next three days the rhythm of questing found its natural flow and I peacefully went through the days, writing my story and paying attention to the nuances and the animals along the way.

By the time Day Three arrived I had recorded a full journal from beginning to end about my breast cancer journey. I also listed the number of animals that I noticed as they visited me on the trip. The first day butterflies danced around the flowers on the steps to my room and then I saw the Javelinas. The Javelinas visited every day and I waited eagerly for their excursion. They felt like my personal pets by the time I left. I also saw the three deer each evening and I spotted one or two more. The second night of my quest I toyed with sleeping on the patio. But in reality I am a big chicken, so I stayed in my room but left the door open with the screen shut and locked. I awakened to a noise on the patio and frightfully got up and checked the outside. There was a huge cat, but it scurried down the patio and climbed into a tree. I could see its long tail dangling and its fiery eyes. This was no ordinary cat or a domestic pet. Staring back at me was a ring-tailed cat, common in the Southern Arizona desert. The next day a fox trotted across the lush green grass below. I wondered if he was looking for the cat.

And what do I make out of those creatures that came to visit me – the snake, the butterfly, the lizard, the deer, the ringtail cat, and the fox? The meaning of each of those spirit visitors can be looked up in various texts. I cannot articulate all of what the animals brought to me, but I chose to view each animal visitor as if it were sent to me during my Vision Quest. For instance, the appearance of the Javelina was clearly one of the best, if not the best, highlight of the quest. They were there to greet me and they appeared often every day throughout my quest. So, what message did the Javelina bring to me? I made the following analogies. Javelina survive in the desert in the weirdest ways. It eats what other animals can't eat. It roots around in the ground for what it needs. It is an animal that lives in community and is good to its young. Part of this quest for me was accepting that I was adding an additional identity to my life. I was now a breast cancer survivor. I ate what others cannot eat by allowing the chemotherapy to rid my body of dangerous cancer cells, I rooted around in the literature and found information useful to myself, and now I was a member of one of the strongest communities in the USA, by participating in the Susan G. Komen Race for the Cure. I also think using my tiger imagery to help me to survive might also qualify as a weird way of surviving amidst my own personal desert.

What did I bring away from the quest? I came home knowing that I needed to write my story. I did that for several months afterward until I became so bogged down in it that I put it away. It has been refreshing to pull it out of the closet and retool it, wrestle with it, and commit it to the printed page. I believe there is a time and season for everything and I knew when I heard it calling from the closet that it was time to finish what the quest had directed me to do.

I wrote this chapter about the quest not only because it is an important part of my story and the key to the writing and publishing of this book but also with the hope that you too, might decide that a suburban rendition of a quest might be helpful to you. I believe each of us should give ourselves time apart to reflect on our life and tweak it in the direction it needs to go. Breast cancer only provided me another opportunity to live well and mindfully, prompting me to take better self-care. Self-care needs to be a part of our everyday ritual and lifestyle, whether we are cancer survivors or not.

CHAPTER 38

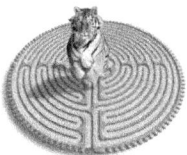

THE F WORD AND A FEW OTHER BOTHERSOME DETAILS

After five years on the drug Tamoxifen, I was supposed to be finished with it. I was so excited about visiting Dr. Langford because I had kept track of the months and days since I began the Tamoxifen. From my perspective, this next appointment in March of 2004 was my five-year mark and the Tamoxifen treatment was supposed to come to an end.

As I sat in my open-to-the-front gown, going over the last six months, the new blood work, etc., Dr. Langford said, "I know you are looking forward to stopping the Tamoxifen. It is time. It has been five years and statistics say it can actually be detrimental to continue after that time."

I noticed he was not finished with his thought. My heart sank as he continued, "However, there is a new drug on the market that will continue to block your estrogen receptors, called Femara. You are the perfect candidate for it and I think it will be a good idea."

Good Idea? This is not *a good idea,* my thoughts rebounded in my head. I just wanted to cry. I was probably as close as I ever was to crying in front of him. Hopes of freedom dashed to the ground. I knew even as my thoughts were swirling that I would take the Femara because of my consistent trust in him, as well as not wanting to miss an important step that might save my life. However, in the back of my mind, I was really ticked. I could not differentiate if I was ticked because I was not yet free, or because of my mistrust in the pharmaceutical industry. Was Femara just another money-making opportunity for them? After all, five years on Tamoxifen might have lined their pockets nicely and saved some lives along the way, but really – another five years?

I quietly tucked my disappointment away, took the prescription, and cried on the way back to my office. "Damn! Will I ever be finished with this treatment?" I lamented.

And, in reality, the answer to that question is "no."

I took the Femara religiously for four years. With each bone density test, my bone density decreased. As a result, I was prescribed the drug Boniva. That was a reluctant decision on my part, since all Boniva does is stop the bone from sloughing off dead cells. Thus, bones become very brittle. Then I had a reaction to Boniva, a reaction that scared me to death. Boniva is prescribed to be taken orally once a month. I took my first dose on a Saturday morning and in the middle of that night I awakened with a fever of 105. Then, three months to the date past my first and only dose of Boniva, I broke out with shingles. The medical field is not sure the two, shingles and Boniva, are related. However, in researching shingles, I understand they can be caused by severe sunburns. My intuition tells me that if shingles can be caused by a bad sunburn then certainly a fever of 105 could be considered an internal bad sunburn. This is a choice point, meaning that I as the patient had to make a medical decision based on personal history, research and probabilities. The correlation fit for me and there was no way that I was going to go back on any similar drug that only keeps my dead cells from sloughing off anyway. Sally Field, the Boniva representative who floods our TV commercials singing the praises of Boniva, is a pleasant woman, but there is nothing she can say that will make me explore another bone density drug. Thus, when I saw my oncologist after the Boniva experience and refused other medications, he looked at his chart and said, "Well, you have been on Femara for four years. Why don't we just stop the drug now? There is no statistically significant difference demonstrated between the four and five year mark."

I was elated. The medical visit was just routine and now I was finally free of the Femara. I made the medical decision at that time, to continue blood work for another year in order to have a record of any changes that might occur as a result of stopping the Femara. That was July 2008. Blood work continued to be within normal range and on March 31, 2010, I was officially discharged from future oncology follow-up appointments. Now *that* really makes me overjoyed.

CHAPTER 39

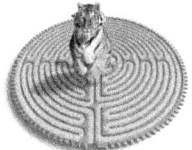

BRINGING CLOSURE

There comes a time and place to bring a good book to an end. My story, however, will continue. Seven years have passed between the pages you just finished reading and this final chapter. A total of eleven years have elapsed since that ominous day in July 1999 when I first discovered my bump. In saying good-bye, I want to punctuate a few things that I think are worth repeating, as well as bring you up to date on my life -----surviving and thriving eleven years later with breast cancer.

Life has continued to be good to me. My private practice has flourished and I am transitioning it to a virtual practice, which means seeing clients through the internet, while maintaining a part-time face-to-face practice. I look forward to seeing clients through the new technology of Skype and presenting workshops on various and sundry topics of interest to others and me. There are many projects and interests that I juggle while I attend to this constant pull to travel and relax. Of course, I want to continue to write, and if you are interested, I have published several self-discovery booklets ready to download from my website at *www.psychotherapyunlimited.com.*

I have also taken risks. Going to the WNBA Fantasy Camp was a big leap out from my comfort zone. Finishing this book is another big leap out of my comfort zone. I plan on continuing to take big bites out of life. I have shed many fears of "I am not good enough" in order to go after my dreams. Even though I may feel small and want to suck my thumb like a child at times, I have learned to tap into my own grace and strength. I am allowing myself to be visible in spite of old beliefs that I don't matter. I am learning that my opinions and beliefs do matter and in my own vulnerability I am finding my strength. Breast Cancer demanded that I be strong.

Living with it. Surviving it.

This year I turned fifty-five, and my story called to me from the darkness of the closet. I knew the time had come to pull the manuscript out of the closet, dust it off, and share my journey. What is it really like when a doctor says to you, "I am sorry, but you have cancer"? Each person who hears those daunting words handles their experience in a unique and personal way. Yet during my journey, I so wanted to hear other people's stories. You have now heard my story and I hope you have found it helpful to you along your journey.

How has my life been different over these past eleven years? Reflecting on that question and posing it to myself, perhaps for the first time. Living with "it" has brought me many gifts, as well as having often haunted me with whispers of fear. What have I learned? Some of what I have learned is hard to capture on paper, but what I can, I will share with you.

Living without Regrets.

Of course, in the past eleven years of living with breast cancer, I also have aged. Life does change with age. This year in particular I found myself looking back at my youth and realized that what I used to do with ease does not come so easily anymore. For instance, I do not remember ever being afraid of heights. But now I have this discomfort with heights and an irrational fear of falling. Perhaps it is that I am no longer immortal as I once thought and my life and time are more precious than ever.

Recently I heard myself telling one of my nieces, "Go to Europe and teach. You are only this age once." As those words echo back to me, I remember and am grateful that in the beginning of my adulthood I traveled to so many places. For me, a child raised in a small mill town in the rural South, I believed that the world began and ended at the Alleghany County line. I know I would have never traveled to California, Hawaii, Australia, New Zealand, Africa or American Samoa if I had not joined a religious group and volunteered several years of my young adult life in Christian ministry.

I look back on those days with gratitude. In some manner the forces in my life saw fit to expel me out of what could have been a rut. I have enjoyed an adventurous life from which I now have so many awesome stories to tell. I am also thankful I was brave enough to accept the challenge of leaving the South, my family of origin, and life as I knew it. Since then, travel has been very important to me. I had been to some wonderful places before cancer. Pam and I have made it a point to travel as much as we can because we enjoy it so much. Traveling is one thing that I believe is different since breast cancer. I am aware that the opportunities to travel are not limitless. We do not put off where we can go today because we are consciously aware we may not be able to go tomorrow. Now, at fifty-five, it has a new twist to it. We say to each other, "Let's go now before we are too old to hike it, explore it, view it, or enjoy it."

Breast cancer has also given me many opportunities to do things differently in my life. Now that I am fifty-five, I look forward to continuing to make changes and do things differently with a great deal of focus and renewed energy. I feel the momentum of moving forward with a new energy. It is as if the autumn of my life has arrived and I want to enjoy the change of season, experiencing fully the vibrant colors and brisk cool air. It is time for new direction, and to re-create myself once again.

Life With My Tiger.

Earlier in this book, I spoke to you of my tiger. My tiger is my daily friend and doorkeeper.   I wear the tiger as a necklace around my neck and continue to practice the ritual of kissing it in the morning and thanking it for doing the work of eating my mutant cells. I believe there is an energy that exists between my tiger and me, and that energy is a mutual sharing of the responsibility to live my life the best I can.

I pay attention to what I eat, my exercise routine, my rest, and my stress. I believe that is how I assist my tiger. I practice gratitude when I kiss and place the necklace mindfully over my head and watch it rest between my breast and my breastlessness. I am grateful. This daily ritual also makes me aware of Don Juan's teaching to Carlos Castaneda in *The Journey to Ixtlan.* As a result of that book, I am mindful that death is always on my shoulder and will counsel me on my life if I turn to it for direction.   During these eleven years, I have had many conversations with death – some poetic and some nakedly scary.

For instance, what if this is my last day? How do I want to spend it? How do I want it to end? I think these are important questions to ask myself from time to time. One exercise I use is to sit quietly with these questions and let the faces of my loved ones pass gently through my mind.   Allowing myself to see their faces and express to them how much I love and care about them makes me aware that I do not want to pass up any opportunity to let them know I love them.   I like this exercise and invite you to try it, too.

Then there are silly thoughts, such as, *Will I ever have another chocolate éclair that tastes this good?* Breast cancer has initiated an array of internal processes and questions about things I always took for granted.

Living With the Whispers of Fear.

I revisit often Carlos Castaneda's book where Don Juan introduces the concept of death as our advisor. I believe that concept is imprinted on my daily psyche. Even though the idea can be romanticized, when I look in the mirror, stare the single-breasted woman in the eye and ask, "Will this get me or will it be something else?" death seems like a very real life consultant.

Whispers of fear echoed each time I had a blood test. Those intrusive whispers became louder and more distinct when my blood test had to be followed by a PET scan. Just recently, my cancer antigen (CA) numbers began to drop a bit. That is a good thing. Perhaps the drop is due to the fact that I have relinquished my unnecessary emotional fight against cholesterol-lowering medication and accepted a prescription for it. I remember Dr. H told me several years ago that statin (cholesterol) medications show some success in helping women with breast cancer because of their anti-inflammatory abilities. I just started taking cholesterol-lowering medication in 2009. And Dr. Langford released me from follow-up oncology appointments on March 31, 2010. I have survived with a passion to live fully and adventurously.

I do not know if our days are numbered before we arrive. I do not know if we only receive a certain number of breaths and then we expire. I do not know if there is a life after death or if there is a heaven or a hell. I realize that, like Castaneda's rabbit, I do not know what Don Juan thinks he knows. I do know that when the time comes, as it will certainly come, I can do nothing to stop it. That is why it is so important to make today, this minute, this instant count. If I am taking my last hop through the dry desert, chewing on beautifully scented purple sage, I do not need to know it is my last meal; but I do need to enjoy it fully and completely as if it is my last meal. If I get to hop another day and visit another bush, then that is a bonus. If not, I would have enjoyed the one from which I last ate.

I do know this one thing for sure – everything in my life can change *In a Moment's Notice.* When I am staring death in the eye, I want to look piercingly with dignity and feel the fear of humanity ending, my humanity. There will always be "what ifs." There will always be stuff in my "in" basket and unfinished projects. I will always have unanswered questions. The goal is to live each day with the questions, and if I live until the answers, that is a good thing; and if I don't, then that is also a good thing.

Each day I tell myself, "Do not hurry. Do not fret. Breathe in and breathe out. Look at the day and decide, where is my passion today? What is important to me today?" After pondering the relevance of that question, I choose how to spend my energy each day.

We each have limitations. We have a limited daily amount of time, energy, and emotional and spiritual resources. I find it is so easy to become baffled or discouraged with all of the things that I wish I could do but do not see any conceivable way of accomplishing. We can become stymied and immobilized if we keep focusing on the pile of things that we think we can't do. If we really can't do something, then we need to drop it and move on to the next. Don't allow yourself to focus on the limits; focus on the possibilities. I encourage you to focus on your resources, your energy, your gifts, and the people in your life and make the most of what you have. Get as close to your goal, your heart, and your passion as you can. Take baby steps daily to make things happen. Sometimes I find that I cannot do something all at once, but if I am patient and continue to gradually move in the direction I want to go, I usually get to where I want to be. And you can too!

Sometimes the analogy between powerful athletes and living each day with a purpose helps me put things into perspective. To be a good athlete, you have to practice. To be an excellent one, you have to practice even more. Winning is exhilarating. To do one's personal best honestly and with integrity I include in my personal values and goals. I know that there is always another race, another competition, and another Super Bowl. I also know that athletes will come and go - some great athletes will make it into the Hall of Fame while others that did not garner as much notoriety count just as much. I have also learned that without the team, there would be no Hall of Fame. I am part of a team and my team is significant to me.

Every person has a story and a personal journey. Her/his story matters to her/him. I encourage you to let your story matter to you. At the end of the day ask yourself, "How pleased am I with myself? What is left unfinished? What will I need to change to become better?"

In my youth, I thought I was invincible. Now, in my fifties, I live with an awareness of my mortality. I am thankful I have been given the gift of eleven more years. I want to be proud of how I live it. I want my story to be told. And I want it to make a difference to you.

Perhaps this manuscript stayed in the closet because one of my biggest fears is that my writing is not good enough? Perhaps it is because I have struggled for so many years with wanting to write and recoiling from the blank page? Perhaps that fear has been more than a whisper, but perhaps another gift of this cancer is my personal need to overcome my fears and write my story anyway.

I would have liked to have waxed strong as a wordsmith and dazzled you with elegance throughout these past pages. I have come to peaceful terms with the fact that this book will bless some and not others. Some will like it, while others will not. Nevertheless, it is my story. Writing it will not make me rich, but I hope it will enrich some lives. My life is richer for having written it.

May yours be richer, too!

Warmly,
Dr. Robin B. Dilley

You may contact me with any questions at my email address: drdilley@psychotherapyunlimited.com

Bibliography

Artress, L. (2006). *Walking a sacred path: Rediscovering the labyrinth as a sacred tool.* New York: The Penguin Group.

Bannerman, H. (1899). *Little black Sambo.* London: Grant Richards Press

Canfield, J. (1993). *Chicken soup for the soul.* NY: Simon and Shuster.

Castaneda, C. (1972). *Journey to Ixtlan.* Roseburg, OR: Simon and Shuster.

Grof, S. (1988). *The adventure of self-discovery.* Albany, NY: SUNY.

Jones, A. (1989). *Soul making: The desert way of spirituality.* San Francisco, CA: Harper Press.

Kaplan, W. S. (1984). *Jungian-Senoi dreamwork manual.* Berkeley, CA: Berkeley Press.

King, S. (1999). *Hearts of Atlantis.* USA: Simon and Shuster.

Kubler-Ross, E. (1973). *Death and dying.* London: Routledge Press.

Love, S. (1990). *Dr. Susan Love's breast health book.* New York: A Merloyd Lawrence Book.

Satir, V. (1988). *The new people making.* Palo Alto, CA: Science and Behavior Books.

Simonton, O. C. (1985). *Getting well again: A step-by-step, self-help guide to overcoming cancer for patients and their families.* Boston, MA:

Shambhala Publications.

Walker, A. (1982). *The color purple.* Orlando, FL: Harcourt. Inc.

About the Author

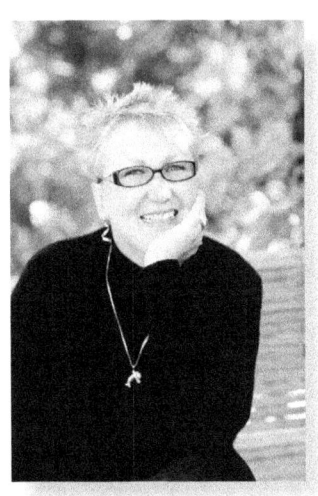

Dr. Robin B. Dilley is a clinical psychologist and a long-term cancer survivor. An acute observer of people, including herself, she is able to capture the essence of situations and then communicate them with clarity, understanding and sensitivity. Her extensive academic and practical background in psychology has been broadened with in-depth study and experience with spirituality and the mind-body-spirit connection.

She has also participated in and taught a variety of spiritual awareness practices. As a result, she has unusually keen insight into the workings of the psyche and how people process life-changing experiences such as a cancer diagnosis and other significant or traumatic events.

Dr. Dilley lives in Phoenix Arizona where she practices, writes, and presents workshops and seminars. Among her most popular presentations are Care of Self-Care of Other, Getting to your Yes, Live Your Life as an Experiment, and others with similarly empowering themes. You can learn more about her through her website, www.inamomentsnotice.com, or follow her on Twitter at www.twitter.com/drrbdilley.

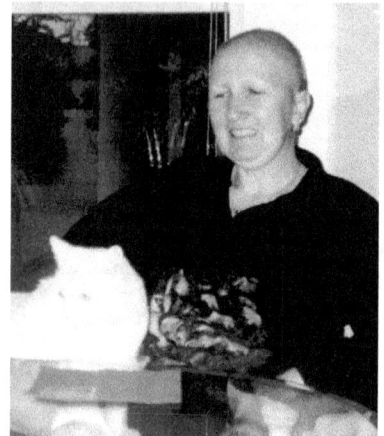

Robin and Schnapps

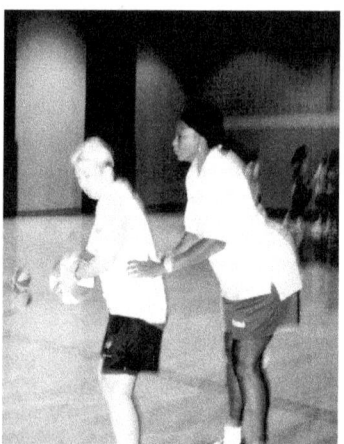

Robin and J. Gillom

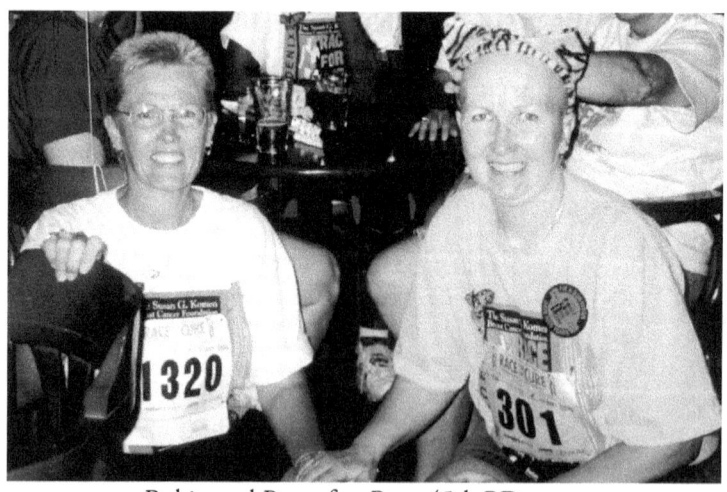

Robin and Pam after Race 45th BD party

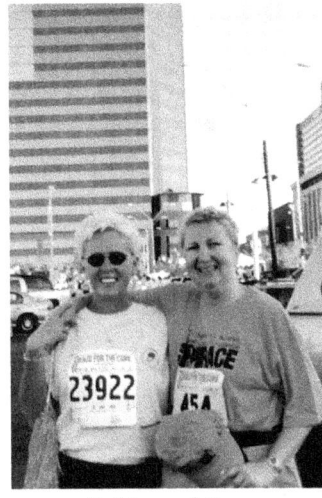

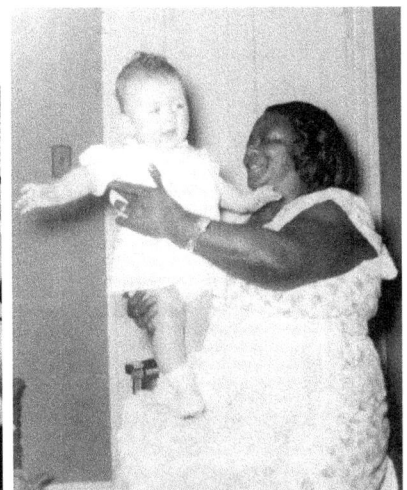

Robin and Pam
Race for the Cure

Baby Robin and Matt

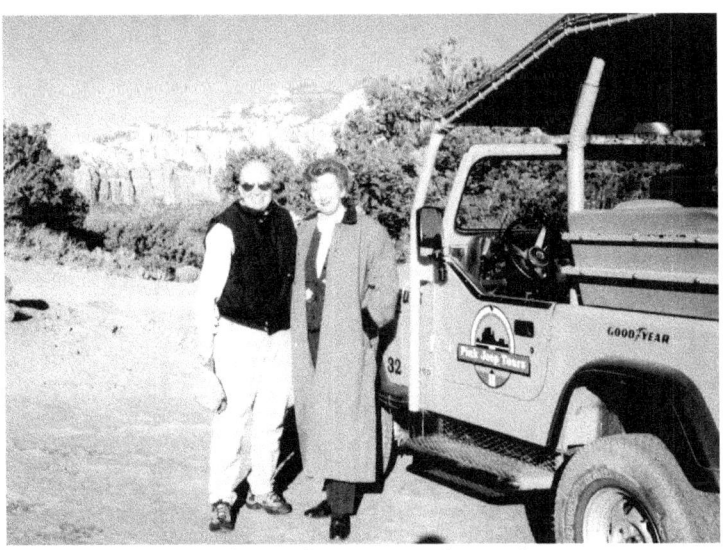

Robin and Cousin Linda Carol

T-Shirt Order

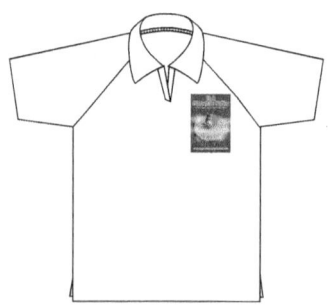

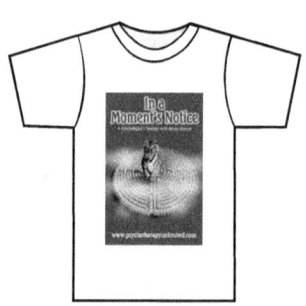

White Polo Style
Short Sleeve Shirt
S-XL = $22.99 + $5.95 s&h
2XL & above = $25.99 + $5.95 s&h

White Short Sleeve T-Shirt
S-XL = $14.99 + $5.95 s&h
2XL & above = $16.99 + $5.95 s&h

White Long Sleeve T-Shirt
S-XL = $17.99 + $5.95 s&h
2XL & above = $19.99 + $5.95 s&h

to order go to

www.allaroundsportsnc.com

All Around Sports of NC, Inc.
7531 S. Va. Dare Trail, Unit 2A
Nags Head, NC 27954
252-449-9002 - office
252-449-9036 - fax

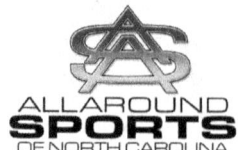

www.ingramcontent.com/pod-product-compliance
Lightning Source LLC
Chambersburg PA
CBHW062139280526
45788CB00001B/225